MEDICAL
ENGLISH
READING

西安交通大学 本科"十四五"规划教材
XI'AN JIAOTONG UNIVERSITY

医学英语系列教材

医学英语阅读教程
·学生用书·

主编 范晓晖 张 鹏
编者 朱 元 彭凤玲 晏国莉
王庆怡 乔玉玲 于 洋

主审 白永权 总主编 陈向京

U0290690

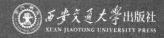

西安交通大学出版社
XI'AN JIAOTONG UNIVERSITY PRESS

Student's Book

图书在版编目（CIP）数据

医学英语阅读教程 / 范晓晖，张鹏主编. —西安：
西安交通大学出版社，2024.9. -- ISBN 978-7-5693
-2017-6

Ⅰ.R

中国国家版本馆CIP数据核字第2024GV5926号

医学英语阅读教程

Medical English · Reading

主　　编	范晓晖　张　鹏
策划编辑	蔡乐芊
责任编辑	蔡乐芊
责任校对	李嫣彧
封面设计	任加盟

出版发行	西安交通大学出版社
	（西安市兴庆南路1号　邮政编码710048）
网　　址	http://www.xjtupress.com
电　　话	（029）82668357 82667874（市场营销中心)
	（029）82668315（总编办）
传　　真	（029）82668280
印　　刷	陕西天意印务有限责任公司

开　　本	787mm×1092mm　1/16　印张　14　字数　410千字
版次印次	2024年9月第1版　2024年9月第1次印刷
书　　号	ISBN 978-7-5693-2017-6
定　　价	45.00元

前　言

医学英语系列教材是一套依据全新的外语教学理念、全新的内容和全新的表达方式编写而成的医学英语教材。该系列教材以教育部新版《大学英语教学指南》为编写指导思想，供医、药、卫生和护理专业本科生教学使用。

全套教材包括《医学英语术语教程》《医学英语阅读教程》和《医学英语视听说教程》三个分册的学生用书和教师用书，共计六本。《医学英语术语教程》可供 36 个学时的教学使用，《医学英语阅读教程》可供 72 个学时的教学使用，《医学英语视听说教程》可供 36 个学时的教学使用。三种教材既自成体系又相互依托，可在教学中单独使用，也可相互组合作为一套系列教材，供 144 个学时的教学使用。

全套教材基本按人体解剖系统分章编写，三种教材均各含 15 章，其中 12 章的主题是相同的。

《医学英语术语教程》是学习医学英语的基础，通过讲解常见医学构词成分来帮助学生快速扩充医学英语词汇量。该教材可为学生学习《医学英语阅读教程》和《医学英语视听说教程》打下基础。

《医学英语阅读教程》旨在培养和提高学生阅读英语医学教科书的能力。每章有两篇阅读文章，内容覆盖该章所讲人体系统的结构、功能和常见病。每篇文章后都配有相关练习。此外，每章最后还配有含思政元素的补充阅读。

《医学英语视听说教程》以提高医学生的医学英语听说能力和医患英语会话技能为宗旨，培养学生理解用英语讲授的医学专业课和用英语进行交流的能力。每章围绕音频或视频材料，设计了丰富多样的视听理解和口语交际活动来提高学生口头表达的能力。

在该套教材的编写过程中，我们获得了众多学校的专家、学者的帮助和支持，在此表示衷心感谢。

总主编

《医学英语阅读教程》编写和使用说明

本书为医学英语系列教材中的《医学英语阅读教程》分册，供医、药、卫生、护理专业本科生教学以及医、药、卫生工作者使用。

1. 编写宗旨

《医学英语阅读教程》旨在通过系统性的、丰富的医学主题阅读，使学生在掌握医学知识的同时，提高其英语阅读能力，打下扎实的医学英语语言基础。

2. 全书框架

本册教材共分 15 章，分别为人体结构与功能概论、细胞与组织、发病机制、骨骼系统、肌肉系统、消化系统、心血管系统、呼吸系统、神经系统、内分泌系统、泌尿系统、淋巴与免疫系统、生殖系统、皮肤系统和感官。

每章由 Pre-Reading Question、Reading 部分的两篇阅读文章和 Medicine in China 以及各部分的相关练习组成。Pre-Reading Question 通过与本章内容相关的谚语及话题导入本章学习内容。Reading 部分包括 Text A 和 Text B，两篇文章的主题相同。以人体某系统为例，Text A 讲解该系统的解剖结构和生理功能，Text B 讲解该系统的常见疾病及其治疗。Medicine in China 为与本章话题相关的含思政元素的文章。通过阅读有关中国医疗卫生政策、我国科研人员取得的前沿医学研究成果、中医治疗及健康生活方式等文章，使学生树立正确的价值观、医学道德和职业操守，增强文化自信，培养国际视野和跨文化交流能力，养成健康的生活方式，在实现英语阅读课程知识目标的同时，使课程思政贯穿教学过程，达到润物无声的效果。

3. 使用说明

1）生词与难点注释：生词的注释包括音标、词性和中文对等词。对课文中的词汇和句法等语言难点都有注释，并通过拓展，举一反三，帮助学生理解和掌握语言知识。

2）每章的两篇课文和生词发音均配有音频，可扫描封底二维码获取。

3）Text A 和 Text B 的练习形式和目的：

• 采用 Multiple-Choice Questions 和 True/False 类练习，考查学生对本章节课文的理解；

• 采用 Matching、Labeling、Grouping 或 Blank Filling 等练习，考查学生对本章节基本词汇的掌握；

• 采用英汉和汉英翻译练习，考查学生的语言运用能力；

• 采用 Summary Writing 练习，要求学生对课文中的某个部分或人体的某个器官的结构或功能进行简述，训练学生的归纳能力及语言综合运用能力；

• 主要采用 Critical Thinking Questions 或 Case Study 任务型学习练习，考查学生学以致用的能力。

4）Medicine in China 的练习形式和目的：

采用段落英译汉和回答问题的练习，考查学生对本部分含思政元素文章的理解及语言应用能力。

本书可供 72 个学时的教学使用。在具体教学中，可根据学生的英语水平和课程时间自由安排。本册配套有相应的教师用书。

在本书的编写过程中，我们获得了众多学校的专家、学者的支持、指导和帮助，在此表示衷心感谢。由于时间紧迫和编者的水平有限，书中难免会存在缺点和错误，望同行和读者不吝赐教。

编者

2024 年 8 月

Contents ◀

Chapter 1   Introduction to the Human Body 1

Text A   Structure and Functions of the Human Body 1

Text B   Factors Affecting Health and Illness 8

"Healthy China 2030" Initiative 14

Chapter 2   Introduction to Cells and Tissues 15

Text A   Cells and Tissues 15

Text B   Cells and Aging 22

China Publishes World's First Stem Cell Related Intl Standard 28

Chapter 3   Introduction to Mechanisms of Diseases 30

Text A   Mechanisms of Diseases 30

Text B   Alzheimer's Disease and Treatment 38

TCM's View of Disease 43

Chapter 4   Skeletal System.. 45

Text A   Structure and Functions of the Skeletal System 45

Text B   Diseases of the Skeletal System and Their Treatment 52

Bionic Bones Strengthen the Future of Orthopedic Implants 57

Chapter 5 Muscular System 58

Text A Structure and Functions of the Muscular System 58

Text B Diseases of the Muscular System and Their Treatment 65

How Can Chinese Medicine Treat Myasthenia Gravis? 71

Chapter 6 Digestive System 72

Text A Structure and Functions of the Digestive System 72

Text B Diseases of the Digestive System and Their Treatment......................... 79

Liver Surgery Pioneer 85

Chapter 7 Cardiovascular System.. 87

Text A Structure and Functions of the Cardiovascular System 87

Text B Diseases of the Cardiovascular System and Their Treatment 94

Tai Chi Good for Your Heart 101

Chapter 8 Respiratory System 103

Text A Structure and Functions of the Respiratory System 103

Text B Diseases of the Respiratory System and Their Treatment 109

TCM Effective in Treating Respiratory Diseases and Cancer 115

Chapter 9 Nervous System 116

Text A Structure and Functions of the Nervous System 116

Text B Diseases of the Nervous System and Their Treatment 124

Brain-Computer Tech on March in Country 131

Chapter 10 Endocrine System... 132

Text A Structure and Functions of the Endocrine System 132

Text B Diseases of the Endocrine System and Their Treatment 139

Eat Healthy Food in Moderation to Help Stay Fit 144

Chapter 11 Urinary System 146

  Text A Structure and Functions of the Urinary System 146

  Text B Diseases of the Urinary System and Their Treatment 152

  Chinese Medical Equipment Transforms Treatment in South Sudan's

  Main Hospital 158

Chapter 12 Lymphatic and Immune System.. 159

  Text A Structure and Functions of the Lymphatic and Immune System 159

  Text B Diseases of the Lymphatic and Immune System and Their Treatment 165

  More Efforts Urged to Curb HIV/AIDS 170

Chapter 13 Reproductive System 172

  Text A Structure and Functions of the Reproductive System 172

  Text B Diseases of the Reproductive System and Their Treatment 179

  Measures to Increase Births Expected to Be Introduced 184

Chapter 14 Integumentary System 186

  Text A Anatomy and Functions of the Integumentary System 186

  Text B Diseases of the Integumentary System and Their Treatment 192

  Appearance Anxiety 197

Chapter 15 Special Senses 199

  Text A Structure and Functions of Special Senses 199

  Text B Diseases of Special Senses and Their Treatment 206

  Auricular Healthcare in TCM 211

Chapter 1

Introduction to the Human Body

Pre-Reading Question

What is the meaning of "in a body"? Is it possible for people to travel in a body?

Reading

Text A Structure and Functions of the Human Body

Human **anatomy** and **physiology** is the study of the structure and function of the human body. The human body consists of many **intricate** parts with **coordinated** functions that are maintained by a complex system of checks and balances. The coordinated function of all the parts of the human body allows us to detect **stimuli**, such as observing a sunset; respond to stimuli, such as removing a hand from a hot object; and perform mental functions, such as remembering and thinking.

Knowledge of the structure and function of the human body allows us to understand how the body responds to a stimulus. For example, eating a candy bar results in an increase in blood sugar (the stimulus). Knowledge of the **pancreas** allows us to predict that the pancreas will **secrete insulin** (the response). Insulin moves into blood **vessels** and is transported to cells, where it increases the movement of sugar from the blood into the cells, providing them with a source of energy. As **glucose** moves into cells, blood sugar levels decrease.

The levels of organization of a language—letters of the **alphabet**, words, sentences, paragraphs, and so on—provide a useful comparison to the levels of organization of the human body. Exploration of the human body will extend from some of the smallest body structures and their functions to the largest structure—an entire person. From the smallest to the largest size of their components, six levels of organization are relevant to understanding anatomy and physiology: the chemical, **cellular**, **tissue**, organ, system, and **organismal** levels of organization (Figure 1-1).

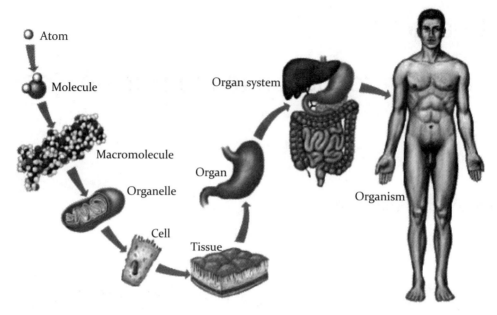

Figure 1-1　Levels of structural organization of the human body

Chemical Level

The structural and functional characteristics of all **organisms** are determined by their chemical makeup. The chemical level of organization involves **interactions** among **atoms** and their combinations into **molecules**. The function of a molecule is related intimately to its structure. For example, **collagen** molecules are strong, ropelike fibers[1] that give skin structural strength and **flexibility**. With old age, the structure of collagen changes, and the skin becomes **fragile** and is torn more easily.

Cellular Level

The cell is the basic structural and functional component of life. Humans are multicellular organisms composed of 60 to 100 **trillion** cells. Although long recognized as the simplest units of the living matter, cells are far from simple. It is at the **microscopic** cellular level that such vital functions of life as **metabolism**, growth, **irritability**, repair, and **replication** are carried out.[2]

Tissue Level

Tissues are groups of cells and materials surrounding them that work together to perform a particular function. There are just four basic types of tissue in your body: **epithelial** tissue, **connective** tissue, muscle tissue, and nervous tissue. An example of a tissue is the heart muscle, whose function is to pump blood through the body.

Organ Level

At the organ level, different kinds of tissues are joined together. Organs are structures that are composed of two or more different types of tissue; they have specific functions and usually have recognizable shapes. Examples of organs are the stomach, heart, liver, lungs, and brain. Figure 1-1 shows how several tissues make up the stomach. The outer covering of the stomach is a layer of epithelial tissue and connective tissue that reduces **friction** when the stomach moves and rubs against other organs. Underneath are the smooth muscle tissue layers, which contract to **churn** and mix food and then push it into the next **digestive** organ, the small **intestine**.[3] The **innermost lining** is an epithelial tissue layer that produces fluid and chemicals responsible for **digestion** in the stomach.

System Level

Systems are the most complex units that make up the body. A system is an organization of varying numbers and kinds of organs that can work together to perform complex functions for the body. For example, the kidneys, the **urinary bladder**, the tubes leading from the kidneys to the bladder, and the tube leading from the bladder to the exterior constitute the urinary system.[4] Sometimes an organ is part of more than one system. The pancreas, for example, is part of both the digestive system and the **hormone**-producing **endocrine** system. There are eleven organ systems in the body.

Organismal Level

The largest organizational level is the organismal level. An organism is any living individual. All the parts of the human body functioning together constitute the total organism—one living person.

The body as a whole is all the atoms, molecules, cells, tissues, organs, and systems. Although capable of being **dissected** or broken down into many parts, the body is a unified and complex **assembly** of structurally and functionally interactive components, all working together to ensure healthy survival.[5]

▶ Word Bank

anatomy /ə'nætəmɪ/ *n.* 解剖；解剖学

intricate /'ɪntrɪkət/ *a.* 错综复杂的

stimulus /'stɪmjʊləs/ *n.* 刺激，刺激物（复数为 stimuli）

pancreas /'pæŋkrɪəs/ *n.* 胰腺

insulin /'ɪnsjʊlɪn/ *n.* 胰岛素

glucose /'gluːkəʊs/ *n.* 葡萄糖

physiology /ˌfɪzɪ'ɒlədʒɪ/ *n.* 生理学

coordinate /kəʊ'ɔːdɪneɪt/ *v.* 协调

secrete /sɪ'kriːt/ *v.* 分泌

vessel /'vesəl/ *n.* 脉管；血管

alphabet /'ælfəbet/ *n.* 字母表

cellular /'seljʊlə/ *a.* 细胞的

tissue /'tɪʃuː/ *n.* 组织

organismal /ˌɔːgə'nɪzməl/ *a.* 有机体的，生物体的

organism /'ɔːgəˌnɪzəm/ *n.* 有机体，生物体

interaction /ˌɪntə'rækʃən/ *n.* 互相影响，互相作用

atom /'ætəm/ *n.* 原子

molecule /'mɒlɪkjʊl/ *n.* 分子

collagen /'kɒlədʒən/ *n.* 胶原，胶原质

flexibility /ˌfleksɪ'bɪlɪtɪ/ *n.* 灵活性；弹性

fragile /'frædʒaɪl/ *a.* 脆的，易碎的

trillion /'trɪljən/ *n.* 万亿，兆

microscopic /ˌmaɪkrə'skɒpɪk/ *a.* 微观的，用显微镜可见的

metabolism /mə'tæbəlɪzəm/ *n.* 新陈代谢

irritability /ˌɪrɪtə'bɪlɪtɪ/ *n.* 应激性

replication /ˌreplɪ'keɪʃən/ *n.* 复制；增殖

epithelial /ˌepɪ'θiːlɪəl/ *a.* 上皮的，皮膜的

connective /kə'nektɪv/ *a.* 连接的；结缔的

friction /'frɪkʃən/ *n.* 摩擦

churn /tʃɜːn/ *v.* 搅拌，搅动

digestive /daɪ'dʒestɪv/ *a.* 消化的；助消化的

intestine /ɪn'testɪn/ *n.* 肠

innermost /'ɪnəˌməʊst/ *a.* 最深处的

lining /'laɪnɪŋ/ *n.* 内层，衬里

digestion /daɪ'dʒestʃən/ *n.* 消化

urinary /'jʊərɪnərɪ/ *a.* 尿的；泌尿的

bladder /'blædə/ *n.* 膀胱

hormone /'hɔːməʊn/ *n.* 激素，荷尔蒙

endocrine /'endəʊkrɪn/ *a.* 内分泌（腺）的

dissect /daɪ'sekt/ *v.* 切开，分开

assembly /ə'semblɪ/ *n.* 集合

▶ Notes

1. ropelike fibers 意为绳状纤维。ropelike 为合成形容词或复合形容词，由 rope（名词）和 like（形容词）构成。合成法（compounding）是英语中常见的构词法，指由两个或更多的词合成新词。用合成法合成的新词称为合成词（compound），这类词在医学英语中相当多，如 hairlike（毛发样的）、flulike（流感样的）。

2. 该句的结构为 It is ... that ... 的强调句型，强调状语 at the microscopic cellular level。本句的正常语序为：Such vital functions of life as metabolism, growth, irritability, repair, and replication are carried out at the microscopic cellular level.。

3. 该句是倒装句。由于主语 the smooth muscle tissue layers 较长，非限定性定语从句如果紧跟在作主语的先行词之后，会造成主语加修饰部分过长，因此需对本句倒装。为了避免重复，underneath 之后省略了前句主语 the outer covering of the stomach。本句的正常语序应为：The smooth muscle tissue layers, which contract to churn and mix food and then push it into the next digestive organ, the small intestine, are underneath the outer covering of the stomach.。

4. 该句中 lead from ... to ... 意为"连接……和……"，the tubes leading from the kidneys to the bladder 指输尿管，the tube leading from the bladder to the exterior 指尿道。两个 leading 分词短语分别为前面名词 the tubes 和 the tube 的定语。

5. 该句中 Although capable of being dissected or broken down into many parts 是让步状语从句，由于从句的主语与主句的主语相同，故省略了从句主语 the body 和系动词 is。all working together to ensure healthy survival 是独立主格结构作伴随状语，all 即 all components。

Exercises

Ⅰ. **Choose the best answer to each of the following questions.**

1. What is the structure of the human body as a whole?
    A. The human body is all the atoms, molecules, cells, tissues, organs, and systems.
    B. The human body mostly consists of atoms, molecules, organs, and systems.
    C. The human body is mainly composed of 60 to 100 trillion cells.
    D. The human body is made up of two or more different types of tissues.

2. The body has multifunctions, which include detecting stimuli, _____.
    A. removing a hand from a hot object, thinking and remembering
    B. coordinating intricate organs and maintaining the balance
    C. maintaining the complexity of the system and producing stimuli
    D. responding to stimuli and performing mental functions

3. An increase in blood sugar by eating a candy bar is used as an example to show _____.
    A. how the body transports insulin
    B. how the body responds to a stimulus
    C. how the body absorbs glucose
    D. how the body provides energy

4. The author makes an analogy (类比) between language and the human body to show that _____.
    A. exploration of the human body is no easier than learning a language
    B. organization of the human body is as complicated as the structure of language
    C. organization of the human body ranges from the smallest to the largest parts
    D. structure of the human body can be divided into six different levels

5. What causes the increased fragility of the skin with old age?
    A. The change of the collagen structure.
    B. The breakdown of the structural strength.
    C. The decrease in the body's flexibility.
    D. The reduction in the amount of collagen.

6. Why are cells still considered important to life, though they are the simplest units of organisms?
    A. Because a vast number of cells exist in the human body.

B. Because vital functions of life can be observed in cells under a microscope.

C. Because cells are living matters and are far from simple.

D. Because many vital functions of life are performed at the cellular level.

7. What is the function of the muscle tissue within the heart?

    A. To pump blood.   B. To protect the heart.

    C. To form the vessel.   D. To transport blood.

8. What are the features that make organs identified easily?

    A. Organs perform complex functions different from those of systems.

    B. Organs are made up of two or more tissues.

    C. Organs have specific functions and recognizable shapes.

    D. Organs are composed of various types of joined tissues.

9. The organismal level is the largest organizational level because _____.

    A. a living human being can be regarded as an organism

    B. all parts of the human body working together make up the organism

    C. an organism can perform the body functions at all levels

    D. an organism is composed of systems which are the most complex units

10. Why do we need to study anatomy and physiology?

    A. To understand the structure and functions of the human body.

    B. To dissect the human body into several parts.

    C. To ensure the healthy survival of human beings.

    D. To understand the human body as an assembly of components.

Ⅱ. **Match each term in Column A with its corresponding description in Column B. Write the corresponding letter in the blank.**

Column A	Column B
_____ 1. anatomy	A. a physical reaction to a specific situation
_____ 2. physiology	B. a thing that causes a specific functional reaction
_____ 3. stimulus	C. the study of body functions
_____ 4. response	D. a hormone produced in the pancreas
_____ 5. insulin	E. the principal circulating sugar in the blood
_____ 6. glucose	F. an individual form of life
_____ 7. tissue	G. a chemical substance that affects how cells and tissues function

_____ 8. organism   H. the process of converting food into chemical substances

_____ 9. hormone   I. a group of similar cells

_____ 10. digestion   J. the study of the structures of the body

Ⅲ. Fill in each blank in the following paragraph with a word in the box. Change the form of words if necessary.

hold	heal	secrete	pancreas	absence
excess	blood	fluid	which	death
maintain	balance	brain	example	recover

The idea that the body 1_____ a balance can be traced back to ancient Greece. It was believed that the body supported four juices: the red juice of 2_____ , the yellow juice of bile, the white juice 3_____ from the nose and lungs, and the black juice in the 4_____ . It was also thought that health resulted from a proper balance of these juices and that disease was caused by a(an) 5_____ of one of them. Normally the body would attempt to 6_____ itself by expelling the excess juice. A(An) 7_____ was the expulsion (排出) of mucus from the nose of a person with a cold, 8_____ led to the practice of bloodletting (放血) to restore the body's normal 9_____ of juices. The practice of bloodletting undoubtedly caused many 10_____ and was eventually abandoned.

Ⅳ. Translate the following English sentences into Chinese.

1. The human body consists of many intricate parts with coordinated functions that are maintained by a complex system of checks and balances.

2. It is at the microscopic cellular level that such vital functions of life as metabolism, growth, irritability, repair, and replication are carried out.

3. Underneath are the smooth muscle tissue layers, which contract to churn and mix food and then push it into the next digestive organ, the small intestine.

4. A system is an organization of varying numbers and kinds of organs that can work together to perform complex functions for the body.

5. Although capable of being dissected or broken down into many parts, the body is a unified and complex assembly of structurally and functionally interactive components, all working together to ensure healthy survival.

Ⅴ. **Write a summary (120w–150w) of Text A.**

Reading

Text B   Factors Affecting Health and Illness

Because health is individually defined by each person and is affected by so many factors, giving a standard definition is difficult. The most widely accepted definition of health was made by the World Health Organization: "Health is a state of complete physical, mental, and social **wellbeing**, not merely the absence of disease or **infirmity**." This definition has expanded since the 1940s, with the development of medical models. On a personal level, most individuals define health according to how they feel ("I feel really sick"), the absence or presence of symptoms of illness ("I have terrible pain in my stomach"), or their ability to carry out activities of daily living ("I felt so much better that I got up and cooked supper").

Illness is also individually defined by each person who experiences an **alteration** in health. It is also difficult to make a standard definition of illness because the terms *disease* and *illness* are often used to mean the same process. Disease is a medical term, meaning that there is a **pathological** change in the structure or function of the body or mind. A disease has specific symptoms and boundaries. An illness, on the other hand, is the response of the person to a disease; it is an abnormal process in which the person's level of functioning is changed compared with a previous level. This response is unique for each person and is influenced by **self-perceptions**, others' perceptions, the effects of changes in body structure and function, the effects of those changes on roles and relationships, and cultural and spiritual values and beliefs. Always remember that a person may have a disease but still achieve **maximum** functioning and quality of life.

Many factors influence a person's health status. These factors may be **internal** or **external** to the individual and may or may not be under the person's conscious control. The factors influencing a person's health-illness status, health beliefs, and health practices relate to the person's health **dimensions**. Each person has these health dimensions, and each dimension influences the behaviors of the person receiving care.

Physical Dimension

The physical dimension includes **genetic inheritance**, age, developmental level, race, and gender. These components strongly influence the person's health status and health practices. As examples, **inherited** genetic disorders include Down syndrome[1], **hemophilia**, **cystic fibrosis**, and color blindness; the **toddler** is at a greater risk for drowning, and the **adolescent** and young adult male are at a greater risk for automobile crashes from excessive speed. There are specific racial traits for disease, including **sickle** cell **anemia**, **hypertension**, and **stroke**. The physical dimension of health could be measured in terms of life **expectancy**[2], the infant **mortality** rate, and other relatively objective measures. However, with advances in technology, particularly in the fields of **imaging**[3] and genetic screening[4], we now recognize that almost all of the populations either have an actual or potential **predisposition** to some future diseases.

Social Dimension

Health practices and beliefs are strongly influenced by a person's economic level, lifestyle, family, and culture. In general, low-income groups are less likely to seek medical care to prevent illnesses, and high-income groups are more **prone** to stress-related habits and illnesses. The family and the culture to which a person belongs influence the person's patterns of living and values about health and illness, which are often **unalterable**. All of these factors are involved in personal care, patterns of eating, lifestyle habits, and emotional stability. Examples of other social-cultural situations that affect health and illness are an adolescent who sees nothing wrong with smoking or drinking because his/her parents smoke and drink, and parents of a sick infant who do not seek medical care because they have no health insurance.

Spiritual Dimension

Spiritual beliefs and values are important components of a person's health and illness behaviors. It is important that care providers respect these values and understand their importance for the individual patient. Measuring the spiritual dimension of health is perhaps the most complex. You would all agree that attendance at places of worship is neither a necessary nor a **sufficient** condition for the full achievement of spiritual health. The absence of crime and violence and the presence of peace and stability in a community where love **prevails** between families and neighbors may be more relevant.

Emotional Dimension

Emotional dimension refers to a person's ability to handle emotions in a constructive way in order to enable him or her to maintain a positive emotional state. Emotional **wellness** helps people achieve positive **self-esteem**, helping them satisfy relationships and providing **resilience** to meet life's challenges. As examples of the negative effects of emotions, a student always has **diarrhea** before examinations and an adolescent with poor self-esteem begins to experiment with drugs. The positive effects of emotions include reducing surgical pain with relaxation techniques and reducing blood pressure with **biofeedback** skills.

Intellectual Dimension

The intellectual dimension **encompasses cognitive** abilities, educational background, and past experiences, which influence a patient's responses to teaching about health and the person's reactions to medical care during illness. They also play a major role in health behaviors. Examples of situations involving these dimensions include the following: An older woman who completed only the fifth grade and needs to be taught how to give herself **injections**; a young college student with **diabetes** who follows a **diabetic** diet but continues to drink beer and eat pizza with friends several times a week; and a middle-aged man who quits taking his high-blood pressure **medication** after developing unpleasant side effects.

It is important to remember that the dimensions **interact** and **overlap**. Changes in one dimension affect the other dimensions. For example, a person who begins an exercise program to lose weight (physical) may also improve his or her self-esteem (emotional). A college student studying philosophy to fulfill university requirements (intellectual) may discover meaning in life and a purpose for living (spiritual). When you have the flu (physical), you probably do not feel like spending time with your friends (social). All in all, health is a state of complete physical, social, and psychological wellbeing that may coexist and interact with illness. Health and illness are viewed as **polar** opposites, but degrees of health and illness are noted from peak wellness to death.

▶ Word Bank

wellbeing /wel'biːɪŋ/ *n.* 幸福，安乐

infirmity /ɪn'fɜːmətɪ/ *n.* 虚弱，衰弱

alteration /ˌɔːltə'reɪʃən/ *n.* 变化

pathological /ˌpæθə'lɒdʒɪkəl/ *a.* 病理学的；病态的

self-perception /ˌselfpə'sepʃən/ *n.* 自我感知

maximum /'mæksɪməm/ *a.* 最高的；最大的

internal /ɪn'tɜːnəl/ *a.* 内部的

external /ɪk'stɜːnəl/ *a.* 外部的

dimension /dɪ'menʃən/ *n.* 维度

genetic /dʒɪ'netɪk/ *a.* 遗传的，基因的

inheritance /ɪn'herɪtəns/ *n.* 继承，遗传

inherit /ɪn'herɪt/ *v.* 继承；遗传而得

hemophilia /ˌhiːmə'fɪlɪə/ *n.* 血友病

cystic /'sɪstɪk/ *a.* 囊的，胞囊的；胆囊的；膀胱的

fibrosis /faɪ'brəʊsɪs/ *n.* 纤维化

toddler /'tɒdlə/ *n.* 学步的小孩

adolescent /ˌædə'lesənt/ *n.* 青少年

sickle /'sɪkl/ *n.* 镰状

anemia /ə'niːmɪə/ *n.* 贫血

hypertension /ˌhaɪpə'tenʃən/ *n.* 高血压

stroke /strəʊk/ *n.* 中风

expectancy /ɪk'spektənsɪ/ *n.* 期望

mortality /mɔː'tælɪtɪ/ *n.* 死亡人数；死亡率

imaging /'ɪmɪdʒɪŋ/ *n.* 成像技术

predisposition /ˌpriːdɪspə'zɪʃən/ *n.* 易染病体质

prone /prəʊn/ *a.* 有……倾向的，易于……的

unalterable /ʌn'ɔːltərəbl/ *a.* 不能改变的

prevail /prɪ'veɪl/ *v.* 盛行

self-esteem /'selfɪs'tiːm/ *n.* 自尊

diarrhea /ˌdaɪə'rɪə/ *n.* 腹泻

intellectual /ˌɪntə'lektʃʊəl/ *a.* 智力的

cognitive /'kɒgnɪtɪv/ *a.* 认知的，认识的

diabetes /ˌdaɪə'biːtiːz/ *n.* 糖尿病

medication /ˌmedɪ'keɪʃən/ *n.* 药物；药物治疗

overlap /ˌəʊvə'læp/ *v.* 重叠

sufficient /sə'fɪʃənt/ *a.* 足够的，充分的

wellness /'welnɪs/ *n.* 健康

resilience /rɪ'zɪlɪəns/ *n.* 弹性，弹力；快速恢复的能力

biofeedback /ˌbaɪəʊ'fiːdbæk/ *n.* 生物反馈

encompass /en'kʌmpəs/ *v.* 包含；包围

injection /ɪn'dʒekʃən/ *n.* 注射

diabetic /ˌdaɪə'betɪk/ *a.* 糖尿病的；适合糖尿病患者的

interact /ˌɪntə'rækt/ *v.* 互相影响，互相作用

polar /'pəʊlə/ *a.* 两极的，正好相反的；极地的

▶ Notes

1.　Down syndrome 意为唐氏综合征（21- 三体综合征，或先天愚型），是由于染色体异常（即多了一条 21 号染色体）而导致的疾病。约 60% 的唐氏综合征患儿早期在胎内即流产，存活者有明显的智力低下、特殊面容、生长发育障碍和多发畸形等症状。

2.　life expectancy 意为预期寿命，是指假设当前的分年龄死亡率保持不变，一个人预期能继续生存的平均年数。预期寿命可以反映出一个社会生活质量的高低。

3.　imaging 意为成像技术。医学影像技术是借助于某种介质（如 X 线、电磁场、超声波、放射性核素等）与人体相互作用，用医学影像学基础理论和技术，把人体内部组织、器官的结构、功能等医疗信息源传给影像信息接收器，最终以影像方式表现出来，供医生诊断疾病。

4.　genetic screening 意为遗传筛查，它是以群体为对象，检测个人是否携带致病基因（通常指隐性遗传病基因），或某种疾病的易感基因型、风险基因型，以防止潜在疾病在个人身上发生或者遗传给后代。遗传筛查可在不同时期、针对不同对象进行。通过遗传筛查，可以尽早发现孩子是否患有先天性遗传病，并及时治疗，使其健康成长。

Exercises

Ⅰ. For each of the following statements, write "T" if the statement is true and "F" if the statement is false in the blank.

_____ 1.　Because health is individually defined by each person, there is no widely accepted definition of health.

_____ 2.　Disease is a medical term which denotes a physical change in the structure of the body.

_____ 3. An illness is an abnormal process in which the person's level of functioning is changed compared with the previous level.

_____ 4. The factors that influence a person's health status are mainly external and not under a person's control.

_____ 5. The physical dimension of health involves genetic inheritance, age, developmental level, race, and sex.

_____ 6. The family and the culture to which people belong have impacts on their lifestyles and values about health.

_____ 7. Living in a safe community filled with love contributes to one's health.

_____ 8. A student who always has diarrhea before examinations is an example of the negative effect of emotion.

_____ 9. The emotional dimension includes cognitive abilities, educational background, and past experiences.

_____ 10. When people have the flu, they probably do not want to spend time with their friends, because the physical dimension might influence the social dimension.

II. **Fill in each blank with a word in the box. Change the form of words if necessary.**

status	spiritual	medication	intake
injection	wellbeing	intellectual	mortality
infirmity	transfusion	cognitive	symptom
syndrome	pathological	genetic	

1. One of the most common _____ of schizophrenia（精神分裂症）is hearing imaginary voices.

2. Another project under way is the use of _____ engineering techniques to develop a vaccine for some diseases.

3. Society expects parents to provide their children with the intimate care that human beings need to develop their _____, emotional, and moral capabilities.

4. On leaving the hospital, the patient felt almost too weak to walk, but he soon overcame this _____.

5. It is absolutely necessary to type the patient's blood before a blood _____.

6. Many factors, which may be internal or external to an individual, influence his or her health _____.

7. Severe acute respiratory _____ (SARS) is a viral respiratory illness caused by a coronavirus (冠状病毒).

8. A new drug delivery system named "nanosponge" (纳米海绵) has shown to be more effective than direct _____.

9. Your doctor will recommend and prescribe specific _____ for pain relief most of the time.

10. People who were physically active on a regular basis had a lower risk of _____ impairments in later life.

Ⅲ. **Translate the following Chinese sentences into English.**

1. 健康是一种身体、心理和社会适应方面都处于完好的状态，而不仅仅是指没有疾病或者不虚弱。

2. 我们应该始终铭记：一个生病的人仍然可以最大限度发挥身体功能，享受高质量的生活。

3. 然而，随着技术进步，特别是在影像和遗传筛查领域的进展，我们现在认识到几乎所有的族群都拥有某种体质，使他们实际或潜在地易患某些疾病。

4. 情绪维度是指人们为保持良好的情绪状态积极应对感情的能力。

5. 虽然健康与疾病被视为对立的两极，但是，从完全健康到死亡之间还存在着各种程度的差异。

Ⅳ. **Think critically and then answer the following questions.**

1. Critics argue that the WHO definition of health is Utopian (乌托邦的), inflexible, and unrealistic, and that including the word "complete" in the definition makes it highly unlikely that anyone would be healthy for a reasonable period of time. It also appears that "a state of complete physical, mental and social well-being" corresponds more to happiness than to health. How do you think of the WHO's definition of health?

2. Health is much more than physical exercise or nutrition. As proposed in Text B, it is the full integration of different states of social, emotional, spiritual, intellectual, and physical wellbeing. What is your opinion about health?

Medicine in China

"Healthy China 2030" Initiative

After the People's Republic of China was founded in 1949, especially since China adopted reform and opening up, the country has made great progress in health-related reforms. Both urban and rural environments have been improved, the Fitness-for-All programs have seen extensive development, sound medical and health service systems have been built, and public health has kept improving. On the other hand, the pace of industrialization, urbanization and aging population, and the changes of the incidences of diseases, ecological conditions and lifestyles are all posing new challenges to China's efforts to maintain and promote people's health, with the provision of healthcare services falling short of increasing demands.

Against such a backdrop, the 18th CPC Central Committee made institutional plans of building a healthy China at its fifth plenary session held in October 2015. In October 2016, the CPC Central Committee and the State Council jointly released an outline for the "Healthy China 2030" initiative, specifying the targets and programs of action. The Party decided to carry out the "Healthy China" initiative at its 19th National Congress, a move to lay a solid foundation for building a prosperous society and turning China into a great modern socialist country that is prosperous, strong, democratic, culturally advanced, harmonious, and beautiful.

Exercises

Ⅰ. **Translate the underlined part into Chinese.**

Ⅱ. **Answer the following question.**

What was the background for the rolling out of the "Healthy China 2030" initiative?

Chapter 2

Introduction to Cells and Tissues

Pre-Reading Question

What is the meaning of "gray cells"? Can we use our gray cells to think?

Reading

Text A   Cells and Tissues

Just as someone who wants to understand buildings must know the building materials, someone who is trying to know the function of the human body must understand cells and tissues. Cells, as the most basic living unit, are at the center of any discussion about the human body. We have trillions of cells, which are organized into different tissues that make up organs, such as our brain, heart, and skin.

Cells

As the basic functional unit of the body, the cell is a highly organized molecular factory. Cells come in a great variety of shapes and sizes. This variation, which is also apparent in sub-cellular structures (**organelles**), reflects the diversity of functions of different cells in the body. All cells, however, have certain features in common such as a cell **membrane**. For descriptive purposes, a cell can be divided into three **principal** parts: cell (**plasma**) membrane, **cytoplasm** and organelles, and **nucleus** (Figure 2-1).

Cell (plasma) membrane: The selectively **permeable** cell membrane gives form to the cell. It controls the **passage** of molecules into and out of the cell and separates the cell's internal structures from the **extracellular** environment.

Cytoplasm and organelles: The cytoplasm is the cellular material between the nucleus and the cell membrane. Organelles are the specialized structures **suspended** within the cytoplasm of the cell that perform specific functions.

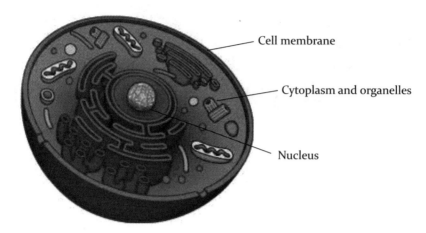

Figure 2-1   Structure of most human cells

Nucleus: The nucleus is the large **spheroid** or **oval** body usually located near the center of the cell. It contains the DNA, or genetic material, that directs the activities of the cell. Within the nucleus, one or more **dense** bodies called **nucleoli** may be seen. The nucleolus contains the **subunits** for **ribosomes**, the structures that serve as sites for protein **synthesis**.

In very general terms, cells perform several basic kinds of work. For example, they **regulate** the **inflow** and **outflow** of materials to ensure that **optimum** conditions for life processes prevail inside the cell. Cells also use their genetic information (DNA) to **ultimately** guide the synthesis of most of their components and direct most of their chemical activities. Among these activities are the **generation** of ATP[1] from the **breakdown** of **nutrients**, synthesis of molecules, transportation of molecules within and between cells, waste removal, and movement of cell parts or even entire cells.[2]

A cell is a complex collection of **compartments**, each of which carries out a host of [3] biochemical reactions that make life possible. However, a cell seldom functions as an isolated unit in the body. They usually work together in groups called tissues.

Tissues

A tissue is a group of similar cells that usually have a common **embryonic** origin and function together to carry out **specialized** activities.[4] The structure and **properties** of a specific tissue are influenced by factors such as the nature of the extracellular material that surrounds the tissue cells and the connections between the cells that compose the tissue. Tissues may be hard, **semisolid**, or even **liquid** in their **consistency**, a range **exemplified** by bone, fat, and blood. In addition, tissues vary **tremendously** with respect to the kinds of cells present, the manner of cell arrangement, and the types of fibers present, if any[5].

Body tissues can be classified into four basic types according to their function and structure: epithelial tissue, connective tissue, muscle tissue, and nervous tissue.

• *Epithelial tissue* may be divided into two types. Covering and lining **epithelium** forms the **epidermis** of the skin and the outer covering of some internal organs. It also forms the inner lining of blood vessels, **ducts**, body **cavities**, and the **interior** of the **respiratory**, digestive, urinary, and **reproductive** systems. **Glandular** epithelium constitutes the secreting portion of **glands**, such as the **thyroid**, **adrenal**, and sweat glands.

• *Connective tissue* is one of the most **abundant** and widely distributed tissues in the body. It binds together, supporting and strengthening other body tissues. It protects and **insulates** internal organs. It **compartmentalizes** structures such as **skeletal** muscles. It is the major transport system within the body (blood is a fluid connective tissue). It is the major site of stored energy **reserves**.

• *Muscle tissue* consists of **elongated** fibers that are beautifully constructed to generate force and produce contraction. As a result of this feature, muscle tissue produces motion, maintains **posture**, and generates heat. Based on its location and structural and functional characteristics, muscle tissue is classified as skeletal, **cardiac**, and smooth.

• *Nervous tissue* is composed of **neurons** which receive and transmit **impulses**, and **neuroglia** which assists in the **propagation** of the nerve impulse as well as in providing nutrients to the neuron. Nervous tissue detects changes in a variety of conditions inside and outside the body and responds by generating nerve impulses. The nervous tissue in the brain helps to maintain **homeostasis**.

Now we know that within the context of a body, cells rarely display **autonomy**. They are so highly specialized in form and function that they have lost the **potential** for independent living, and are often **clustered** into clearly **identifiable** masses—tissues.[6] Each organ actually has a mixture of different tissues within it. These tissues are arranged in ways that allow the organ to carry out its functions. Some of the tissues actually do the work of that organ while others are there to support those tissues doing that work.

▶ **Word Bank**

organelle /ˌɔːgə'nel/ *n.* 细胞器　　　　membrane /'membreɪn/ *n.* 膜，薄膜

principal /'prɪnsəpəl/ *a.* 主要的　　　　plasma /'plæzmə/ *n.* 血浆

cytoplasm /'saɪtəʊˌplæzəm/ *n.* 细胞质　　nucleus /'njuːklɪəs/ *n.* 核仁；神经核

permeable /'pɜ:mɪəbl/ *a.* 有渗透性的

extracellular /ˌekstrə'seljʊlə/ *a.* 细胞外的

spheroid /'sfɪərɔɪd/ *a.* 球状的

dense /dens/ *a.* 稠密的

subunit /'sʌbju:nɪt/ *n.* 亚单位

synthesis /'sɪnθɪsɪs/ *n.* 合成

inflow /'ɪnfləʊ/ *n.* 流入

optimum /'ɒptɪməm/ *a.* 最佳的

generation /ˌdʒenə'reɪʃən/ *n.* 产生

nutrient /'nju:trɪənt/ *n.* 营养物质

embryonic /ˌembrɪ'ɒnɪk/ *a.* 胚胎的

property /'prɒpətɪ/ *n.* 性质，特性

liquid /'lɪkwɪd/ *a.* 液体的

exemplify /ɪg'zemplɪfaɪ/ *v.* 例证

epithelium /ˌepɪ'θi:lɪəm/ *n.* 上皮

duct /dʌkt/ *n.* 导管

interior /ɪn'tɪərɪə/ *n.* 内部

reproductive /ˌri:prə'dʌktɪv/ *a.* 生殖的

gland /glænd/ *n.* 腺

adrenal /ə'dri:nəl/ *a.* 肾上腺的

insulate /'ɪnsjʊleɪt/ *v.* 使绝缘；隔离

skeletal /'skelɪtəl/ *a.* 骨骼的

elongated /ɪ'lɔ:ŋgeɪtɪd/ *a.* 细长的

cardiac /'kɑ:dɪæk/ *a.* 心脏的；贲门的

impulse /'ɪmpʌls/ *n.* 冲动；（电）脉冲

propagation /ˌprɒpə'geɪʃən/ *n.* 传播

autonomy /ɔ:'tɒnəmɪ/ *n.* 自主，独立

cluster /'klʌstə/ *v.* 簇集

passage /'pæsɪdʒ/ *n.* 通过；通路

suspend /sə'spend/ *v.* 悬浮

oval /'əʊvəl/ *a.* 卵形的

nucleolus /ˌnjuklɪ'əʊləs/ *n.* 核仁（复数为 nucleoli）

ribosome /'raɪbəsəʊm/ *n.* 核糖体

regulate /'regjʊleɪt/ *v.* 调节

outflow /'aʊtfləʊ/ *n.* 流出

ultimately /'ʌltɪmətlɪ/ *ad.* 最后，最终

breakdown /'breɪkdaʊn/ *n.* 分解

compartment /kəm'pɑ:tmənt/ *n.* 隔间

specialized /'speʃəlaɪzd/ *a.* 专门的

semisolid /ˌsemɪ'sɒlɪd/ *a.* 半固体的

consistency /kən'sɪstənsɪ/ *n.* 稠度

tremendously /trɪ'mendəslɪ/ *ad.* 非常地

epidermis /ˌepɪ'dɜ:mɪs/ *n.* 表皮

cavity /'kævɪtɪ/ *n.* 腔；洞

respiratory /'respərətərɪ/ *a.* 呼吸的

glandular /'glændjʊlə/ *a.* 腺的；起腺体功能的

thyroid /'θaɪrɔɪd/ *a.* 甲状腺的

abundant /ə'bʌndənt/ *a.* 丰富的

compartmentalize /ˌkɒmpɑ:t'mentəlaɪz/ *v.* 划分；区分

reserve /rɪ'zɜ:v/ *n.* 储量

posture /'pɒstʃə/ *n.* 姿势

neuron /'njʊərɒn/ *n.* 神经元

neuroglia /ˌnjʊə'rɒglɪə/ *n.* 神经胶质

homeostasis /ˌhɒmɪə'steɪsɪs/ *n.* 体内稳定，体内稳态

potential /pə'tenʃəl/ *n.* 潜能

identifiable /aɪ'dentɪˌfaɪəbl/ *a.* 可辨认的

▶ Notes

1. ATP 意为三磷酸腺苷，为 adenosine triphosphate 的缩写，它是人体内一切生命活动所需能量的直接来源。

2. 该句为倒装句式，为承接上句中的 chemical activities，保持句子连贯，避免主语过长，而将表语放在句首。

3. a host of 意为一大群，许多，该短语一般修饰可数名词。例如：Lead toxicity causes a host of surprisingly unpleasant health conditions.。

4. 该句的结构较复杂：The structure and properties of a specific tissue are influenced by factors 为该句主干，such as 后面连接了两个名词短语，分别是 the nature of

the extracellular material that surrounds the tissue cells 和 the connection between the cells that compose the tissue；名词短语中的两个 that 引导的定语从句，分别修饰先行词 the extracellular material 和 the cells。

5. if any 意为果真有或即使有的话，起到加强语气的作用。例如：Please correct mistakes, if any.。

6. 该句为 so ... that 句型，其中 that 引导的结果状语从句包含并列谓语 have lost the potential for independent living 和 are often clustered into clearly identifiable masses—tissues 两个部分；破折号起解释和强调作用，即 tissues 指 clearly identifiable masses。

Exercises

Ⅰ. Choose the best answer to each of the following questions.

1. What is the relation between cells and tissues?
   A. Similar cells make up a tissue.
   B. Cells are far more important than tissues.
   C. The structure of cells is determined by tissues.
   D. The function of cells is related to the structure of tissues.

2. A cell can be divided into cell membrane, nucleus, and _____.
   A. plasma and cytoplasm
   B. cytoplasm and organelles
   C. atoms and molecules
   D. proteins and DNA

3. According to the passage, cells are different in shape and size because of _____.
   A. the diversity of cytoplasm in cells
   B. the typical features that cells share
   C. their different functions in the body
   D. the different number of molecules in cells

4. What function does the cell membrane perform?
   A. It gives shape to the cell and controls the passage of molecules.
   B. It directs cells' activities and provides sites for protein synthesis.
   C. It generates DNA and maintains the structure of cells.
   D. It reflects the diversity of cells and controls the flow of organelles.

5. Which one of the following is a basic function of cells?
   A. Protecting and insulating the organs.

B. Creating balanced conditions for life processes.

C. Guiding the synthesis of their components.

D. Generating heat in the human body.

6. What factor(s) influence(s) the structure and traits of a certain tissue?

A. The way the extracellular material surrounds the cells.

B. The number of cells that work together to form the tissue.

C. The biochemical reactions that take place in the cells.

D. The nature of the material outside cells and the links between the cells.

7. The epithelial tissue can be classified into glandular epithelium and

_____.

A. outer covering epithelium   B. inner lining epithelium

C. covering and lining epithelium   D. epidermis of the skin

8. Which type of tissue is among the most widely distributed tissues in the body?

A. Epithelial tissue.   B. Connective tissue.

C. Muscle tissue.   D. Nervous tissue.

9. According to the passage, muscle tissue can _____.

A. generate force and create contraction

B. compartmentalize structures and produce motion

C. maintain gestures and provide nutrients

D. store energy and detect impulses

10. Why can't cells live independently?

A. Because they often cluster into clearly recognizable groups.

B. Because they need to maintain the homeostasis in the body.

C. Because they live in the context of the body.

D. Because they have their specialized form and function.

Ⅱ. **Fill in each blank with a proper word mentioned in the text. The first letter of the word is given.**

1. The cell m_____ forms a barrier between the inside of the cell and the outside, so that the chemical environments on the two sides can be different.

2. As the cellular factories that make proteins, r_____ are essential for life in organisms ranging from bacteria to humans.

3. The n_____, located in the center of a cell, contains the genetic material DNA.

4. The group of cells that maintains the form of organs and provides internal support in the body is known as the c_____ tissue.

5. Cells use their DNA to guide the s_____ of most of their components and direct most of their chemical activities.

6. Glandular e_____ constitutes the secreting portion of glands such as the thyroid and adrenal glands.

7. In cell biology, molecular biology, and related fields, the word e_____ means "outside the cell".

8. Digestion is the b_____ of food into smaller particles or individual nutrients, with the help of several body fluids.

9. A chemical r_____ is a process in which one substance is converted to another substance.

10. When n_____ tissue detects a change in conditions outside the body, it produces nerve impulses.

Ⅲ. Fill in each blank in the following paragraph with a word in the box. Change the form of words if necessary.

end	answer	sign	gene	other
result	another	specialize	differentiate	shape
cause	biology	cell	signal	tissue

Each human organism begins as a single 1_____, a fertilized egg, which divides to create two cells, each of which divides in turn, 2_____ in four cells, and so on. If cell multiplication (增殖) were the only event occurring, the 3_____ result would be a spherical (球形的) mass of identical cells. The process of transforming an unspecialized cell into a 4_____ cell is known as cell differentiation (分化), the study of which is one of the most exciting areas in 5_____ today. All cells in a person have the same 6_____; how then is one unspecialized cell instructed to 7_____ into a nerve cell, 8_____ into a muscle cell, and so on? What are the external chemical 9_____ that constitute these "instructions," and how do they affect various cells differently? The 10_____ to these questions are unknown.

Ⅳ. **Translate the following English sentences into Chinese.**

1. Just as someone who wants to understand buildings must know the building materials, someone who is trying to know the function of the human body must understand cells and tissues.

2. Cell membrane controls the passage of molecules into and out of the cell and separates the cell's internal structures from the extracellular environment.

3. A cell is a complex collection of compartments, each of which carries out a host of biochemical reactions that make life possible.

4. Tissues vary tremendously with respect to the kinds of cells present, the manner of cell arrangement, and the types of fibers present.

5. Nervous tissue is composed of neurons which receive and transmit impulses, and neuroglia which assists in the propagation of the nerve impulse as well as in providing nutrients to the neuron.

Ⅴ. **Write a summary (120w–150w) of Text A.**

Reading

Text B   Cells and Aging

Have you ever wondered why we age? What exactly is happening inside our bodies that brings on the **wrinkles**, gray hair, and other changes seen in older people? Considering the **universality** of the process, you might be surprised to know that there remain many unanswered questions about how aging happens at the cellular level. However, theories **abound**, and the roles played by various **suspects** in the aging process are beginning to take shape.

Scientists all agree that different cells have different replication capabilities and life spans. Some cells, such as those that line the **gastrointestinal** tract, reproduce continuously. Some other cells, such as the cells on the inside of **arteries**, lie **dormant** but are capable of replicating in response to injury. Those cells which cannot reproduce include cells of the heart, nerves, and muscles, some of which have short life spans and must be continually replaced by other cells in the body (Red and white blood cells are examples.).[1] Others, such as heart and nerve cells, live for years or even decades. Over time, cell death **outpaces** cell production, leaving us with fewer cells. As a result, we are less capable of repairing wear and tear[2] on the body, and our **immune** system is **compromised**. We become more **susceptible** to[3] **infections** and less **proficient** at seeking out and destroying **mutant** cells that could cause **cancerous** tumors. In fact, many older adults **succumb** to conditions that they could have resisted in their youth.[4]

Evidence is **mounting** to support the **hypothesis** that stress, in the form of **toxic oxidants**, as well as other DNA-damaging **agents** produced by our cells and the environment (**radiation**, smoke, and toxic metals), can **induce** cellular **senescence**. Free **radicals** produce damage in **lipids**, proteins or **nucleic** acids and result in wrinkled skin, stiff **joints**, and hardened arteries. Normal cellular metabolism such as **aerobic** cellular **respiration** in **mitochondria** produces some free radicals. Others are present in air pollution, radiation, and certain foods we eat.

Glucose, the most abundant sugar in the body, is another factor that plays a role in the aging process. It is **haphazardly** added to proteins inside and outside cells, forming **irreversible** cross-links between **adjacent** protein molecules. With advancing age, more cross-links form, which contributes to the stiffening and loss of **elasticity** that occur in aging tissues.

Furthermore, cellular senescence can result from the overproduction of certain **regulators** (**oncogenes**) of cell **division**. These oncogenes, too, can be **activated** by cell stress-inducing toxic agents. These forms of stress do not involve **telomere** shortening, yet can cause a cell to **senesce** in a relatively short period of time.

While some theories of aging explain the causes of aging, others concentrate on **mechanisms** operating at the cellular level. DNA damage, decreased cellular replication, and **defective** protein homeostasis are thought to be the mechanisms responsible for cellular aging.

DNA damage is an alteration in the structure of DNA. A variety of metabolic **insults** that **accumulate** over time may result in damage to nuclear and **mitochondrial** DNA. Although most DNA damage is repaired by DNA repair **enzymes**, some damage persists and accumulates as cells age. Some aging syndromes are associated with defects in DNA repair mechanisms, and the life span of experimental animals in some models can be increased if responses to DNA damage are enhanced or proteins that **stabilize** DNA are introduced.[5]

Decreased cellular replication refers to the limited **capacity** of cells for replication. After a fixed number of divisions, cells become **arrested** in a **terminally** nondividing state, known as **replicative** senescence. Aging is associated with progressive replicative senescence of cells. Cells from children have the capacity to **undergo** more rounds of replication than do cells from older people. In contrast, cells from patients with **Werner syndrome**[6], a rare disease characterized by **premature** aging, have a **markedly** reduced **in vitro** life span.

Defective protein homeostasis happens when cells are unable to maintain normal protein homeostasis, because of increased **degradation** and decreased synthesis caused by reduced **translation** of proteins and defective activity of **chaperones** (which promote normal protein folding), **proteasomes** (which destroy misfolded proteins), and repair enzymes. Abnormal protein homeostasis can have many effects on cell survival, replication, and functions. In addition, it may lead to the accumulation of misfolded proteins, which can **trigger** pathways of **apoptosis**.

No matter how the theories vary, one thing we cannot deny is that all cells experience changes with aging. In this process, cells become larger and are less able to divide and **multiply**, and eventually lose their ability to function or begin to function abnormally. In technical terms, cell aging is the result of a progressive decline in cellular function and **viability** caused by genetic **abnormalities** and the accumulation of cellular and molecular damage due to the effects of exposure to **exogenous** influences.[7] Understanding cell aging **propels** our ability to treat diseases, such as cancer, heart disease, **Alzheimer's disease**, **malaria**, **tuberculosis**, and AIDS, and can help us prepare for new diseases.

▶ **Word Bank**

wrinkle /'rɪŋkl/ *n.* 皱纹

abound /ə'baʊnd/ *v.* 丰富，充满

gastrointestinal /ˌɡæstrəʊɪn'testɪnəl/ *a.* 胃肠的

dormant /'dɔ:mənt/ *a.* 静止的

immune /ɪ'mju:n/ *a.* 免疫的；有免疫力的

susceptible /sə'septɪbl/ *a.* 易受……影响的；易受（伤）的；易患（病）的

infection /ɪn'fekʃən/ *n.* 感染

mutant /'mju:tənt/ *a.* 突变的

succumb /sə'kʌm/ *v.* 死；被压垮

hypothesis /haɪ'pɒθɪsɪs/ *n.* 假设，假说

oxidant /'ɒksɪdənt/ *n.* 氧化剂

radiation /ˌreɪdɪ'eɪʃən/ *n.* 辐射；放射物

senescence /sɪ'nesəns/ *n.* 衰老

lipid /'lɪpɪd/ *n.* 脂质

joint /dʒɒɪnt/ *n.* 关节

respiration /ˌrespɪ'reɪʃən/ *n.* 呼吸

mitochondrion /ˌmaɪtəʊ'kɒndrɪən/ *n.* 线粒体（复数为 mitochondria）

haphazardly /hæp'hæzədlɪ/ *ad.* 随意地

adjacent /ə'dʒeɪsənt/ *a.* 邻近的

regulator /'reɡjʊleɪtə/ *n.* 调控者；调节因子

division /dɪ'vɪʒən/ *n.* 分裂

universality /ˌju:nɪvɜ:'sælətɪ/ *n.* 普遍性

suspect /'sʌspekt/ *n.* 怀疑，嫌疑；可疑对象

artery /'ɑ:tərɪ/ *n.* 动脉

outpace /aʊt'peɪs/ *v.* 速度超越

compromise /'kɒmprəmaɪz/ *v.* 损害，危害

proficient /prə'fɪʃənt/ *a.* 熟练的，精通的

cancerous /'kænsərəs/ *a.* 癌的，癌变的

mount /'maʊnt/ *v.* 增加，上升；发动

toxic /'tɒksɪk/ *a.* 有毒的

agent /'eɪdʒənt/ *n.* 因子；药剂

induce /ɪn'dju:s/ *v.* 引起，诱发

radical /'rædɪkəl/ *n.* 原子团，基

nucleic /nju:'kli:ɪk/ *a.* 核的

aerobic /eə'rəʊbɪk/ *a.* 需氧的

irreversible /ˌɪrɪ'vɜ:sɪbl/ *a.* 不可逆的

elasticity /ˌɪlæ'stɪsɪtɪ/ *n.* 弹力；弹性

oncogene /'ɒŋkəʊdʒi:n/ *n.* 致癌基因

activate /'æktɪveɪt/ *v.* 激活，使活动

telomere /'teləmɪə/ *n.* 端粒

mechanism /'mekəˌnɪzəm/ *n.* 机制，机理

insult /'ɪnsʌlt/ *n.* 损伤

mitochondrial /ˌmaɪtəʊ'kɒndrɪəl/ *a.* 线粒体的

stabilize /'steɪbəlaɪz/ *v.* 使稳定

arrest /ə'rest/ *v.* 阻止，遏止

replicative /'replɪkeɪtɪv/ *a.* 复制的

Werner syndrome /'wɜːnə 'sɪndrəʊm/ 沃纳综合征

premature /ˌprɪmə'tjʊə/ *a.* 早熟的；早产的

in vitro /ɪn ɪn'viːtrəʊ/ *ad.* 在试管内，体外

translation /træns'leɪʃən/ *n.* 转变，转化

proteasome /ˌprəʊti:'sɒm/ *n.* 蛋白酶体

apoptosis /ˌæpəp'təʊsɪs/ *n.* 细胞凋亡

viability /ˌvaɪə'bɪlətɪ/ *n.* 生存力，活力；发育能力

exogenous /ek'sɒdʒənəs/ *a.* 外因的；外源的

Alzheimer's disease /ˈæl'zeməz dɪ'zi:z/ *n.* 阿尔茨海默病，老年痴呆

malaria /mə'leərɪə/ *n.* 疟疾

senesce /'senəs/ *v.* 开始衰老

defective /dɪ'fektɪv/ *a.* 有缺陷的

accumulate /ə'kju:mjʊleɪt/ *v.* 累积，积聚

enzyme /'enzaɪm/ *n.* 酶

capacity /kə'pæsɪtɪ/ *n.* 能力

terminally /'tɜːmɪnəlɪ/ *ad.* 末期地

undergo /ˌʌndə'gəʊ/ *v.* 经历

markedly /'mɑːkɪdlɪ/ *ad.* 明显地

degradation /ˌdegrə'deɪʃən/ *n.* 退化

chaperone /'ʃæpərəʊn/ *n.* 分子伴侣

trigger /'trɪgə/ *v.* 引发，触发

multiply /'mʌltɪplaɪ/ *v.* 增加

abnormality /ˌæbnɔ:'mælɪtɪ/ *n.* 异常

propel /prə'pel/ *v.* 推进，驱使

tuberculosis /tjʊˌbɜːkjʊ'ləʊsɪs/ *n.* 肺结核

▶ Notes

1.　该句主句为 those cells include cells of the heart, nerves, and muscles。限定性定语从句 which cannot reproduce 修饰先行词 cells。非限定性定语从句 some of which have short life spans and must be continually replaced by other cells in the body 中 which 指代 include 后的 cells。

2.　wear and tear 意为磨损。wear and tear 是固定搭配的名词词组，常用于生物和机械领域，表示耗损或磨损，例如：Your gums may also be showing some wear and tear from too much chewing.。

3.　become susceptible to 意为易患病的。susceptible 通常指易受影响的，例如：Young people are the most susceptible to advertisements.。在医学用语中，它通常表示易患病的，例如：Walking with weights makes the shoulders very susceptible to injury.。

4.　该句为复合句，定语从句中 could have resisted 为虚拟语气，在此语境中表示纯粹的假设。could have done 还可以表示本来能够做某事而没有做，如：He could have passed the exam, but he was too careless.。

5.　该句为并列复合句。and 前后为并列成分。后半部分又包含 if 引导的条件状语从句，连词 or 连接两个条件状语从句 responses to DNA damage are enhanced 和 proteins that stabilize DNA are introduced。

6.　Werner syndrome，沃纳综合征，也称早老症，是一种先天性常染色体隐性遗

传性疾病，多见于有血缘婚姻的子代，尤以堂兄妹间结婚者的子代居多。该病的主要特征包括老人样面容、身材矮小、青少年白发、青年白内障、四肢硬皮病样皮肤改变、骨质疏松、组织钙化、糖尿病和性腺发育不全等。

7. 该句的主干为 cell aging is the result of a progressive decline in cellular function and viability。过去分词短语 caused by genetic abnormalities and the accumulation of cellular and molecular damage 作定语修饰 decline，形容词短语 due to the effects of exposure to exogenous influences 作定语修饰 the accumulation of cellular and molecular damage。

Exercises

Ⅰ. **For each of the following statements, write "T" if the statement is true and "F" if the statement is false in the blank.**

_____ 1. Researchers have understood how aging happens at the cellular level.

_____ 2. Although the life spans of cells vary according to their types, cells have the same replication capabilities.

_____ 3. Heart cells and nerve cells cannot reproduce, but they can live for a very long time.

_____ 4. Glucose interacts with the proteins inside the cells only, forming unalterable links between molecules.

_____ 5. Glucose, free radicals, and oncogenes may result in the aging of cells.

_____ 6. DNA damage refers to the changes occurring in the structure of DNA.

_____ 7. Patients with Werner syndrome experience premature aging because their cells' replication capability is greater than usual.

_____ 8. Abnormal protein homeostasis may cause the accumulation of miscoded proteins and activate the pathway of apoptosis.

_____ 9. Some researchers insist that some of the cells experience no changes with aging.

_____ 10. DNA damage, decreased cellular replication, and defective protein homeostasis are considered as factors affecting cellular aging.

Ⅱ. Match each term in Column A with its corresponding description in Column B. Write the corresponding letter in the blank.

Column A	Column B
_____ 1. aging	A. a process by which DNA makes a copy of itself
_____ 2. wrinkle	B. the change of something from one phase to another
_____ 3. senescence	C. a theory that is not yet verified
_____ 4. replication	D. an increase by natural growth or addition
_____ 5. hypothesis	E. energy that is transmitted in the form of rays
_____ 6. radiation	F. a process that occurs during the chemical reaction
_____ 7. viability	G. the capability of surviving
_____ 8. alteration	H. the organic process of growing older
_____ 9. accumulation	I. line on the surface of the skin
_____ 10. division	J. the process of growing older

Ⅲ. Translate the following Chinese sentences into English.

1. 不管怎样，关于衰老有诸多理论，各种疑似因素在衰老过程中的作用机制也逐渐被认识清楚。

2. 随着时间的推移，细胞死亡速度超过再生速度，体内细胞就会减少。

3. 越来越多的事实支持这种假说：以毒性氧化物形式出现的应激以及由细胞与环境（辐射、烟雾和有毒金属）导致的其他脱氧核糖核酸损伤因子会诱发细胞衰老。

4. 脱氧核糖核酸损伤、细胞增殖减少、蛋白平衡缺陷都被认为是造成细胞衰老的机制。

5. 了解细胞衰老有助于我们提高治疗诸如癌症、心脏病、阿尔茨海默病、疟疾、肺结核、艾滋病等疾病的能力，也能帮助我们为应对新疾病作好准备。

Ⅳ. Think critically and then answer the following questions.

1. Understanding the determinants of cellular aging is critical to the understanding of human longevity. In Text B, six factors that might cause the aging of cells are mentioned. Some researchers believe if we can eliminate these factors that cause cell aging, humans can live eternally. Do you think it is a fancy dream or it can come true one day?

2. Empirical（实证的）evidence shows that normal human cells in a cell culture will divide about 50 times and then enter the phase of cell death. Take skin as an example. Totally 30,000 to 40,000 skin cells die every minute, which means we lose around 50 million cells every day. Can you explain how cell death causes the loss of elasticity and wrinkles in our skin?

Medicine in China

China Publishes World's First Stem Cell Related Intl Standard

China published the world's first international standard on stem cell research in September 2022, signaling that the country has become a globally recognized front-runner in this cutting-edge field that may revolutionize medicine, experts said.

The document, named ISO 24603, lists the various requirements and regulations for cultivating and using human and mouse pluripotent stem cells. It is also the first stem cell-related standard for the International Organization for Standardization.

Pluripotent stem cells have the ability to differentiate into any cell types that make up the body. They are typically found during the earliest stages of cell division after fertilization. As a result, scientists are trying to harness the regenerative potential of stem cells to treat many challenging medical conditions, such as spinal cord injuries, leukemia, type 1 diabetes, heart diseases, stroke, burns, Alzheimer's disease, and Parkinson's disease, according to the Mayo Clinic.

However, stem cell therapy can be controversial due to it being poorly regulated, with unscrupulous providers hyping the technology and drawing patients seeking cures to illegal and potentially harmful treatments.

Chen Yeguang, the president of the Chinese Society for Cell Biology, said stem cell and regenerative medicine is a rapidly developing field, and it is essential to build consensus and establish some ground rules for research and the industry. "ISO 24603 will play an extremely important role in setting standards for the whole industry and public health," he said.

Zheng Jian, deputy director of the Department of Basic Research of the Ministry of Science and Technology, said the standard not only provides crucial instructions to guide and support the development of the stem cell industry but also showcases China's increased international recognition in stem cell research. "It has injected positive energy into China's science, technology, and innovation in life and health sciences," he said.

Exercises

Ⅰ. **Translate the underlined part into Chinese.**

Ⅱ. **Answer the following question.**

What was the significance for China to publish the first stem cell-related standard for the International Organization for Standardization?

Chapter 3

Introduction to Mechanisms of Diseases

Pre-Reading Question

What is the meaning of "a foot-in-mouth disease"? Have you seen anyone with a foot-in-mouth disease?

Reading

Text A   Mechanisms of Diseases

Disease can be broadly described as an abnormality in body function that threatens a person's wellbeing. Mechanisms of disease reveal the functional and structural changes in disease from the molecular level to the effects on the individual.[1] To gain a better understanding of the different mechanisms of disease, scientists usually study the causes of diseases, which are commonly divided into six categories: genetic disorder, **trauma**, **inflammation**, infection, **neoplasm**, and **impaired immunity**.

Genetic Disorder

Genetic disorder is caused by an alteration of an individual's genetic or **chromosomal** makeup. Based on their genetic contribution, human diseases can be classified as **monogenic**, chromosomal, or **multifactorial**. Monogenic diseases are caused by alterations in a single gene, and they **segregate** in families according to the traditional **Mendelian** principles of inheritance. Chromosomal diseases, as their name indicates, are caused by alterations in **chromosomes**. For instance, within an individual's **genome**, some chromosomes may be missing, extra chromosome copies may be present, or certain portions of chromosomes may be deleted or **duplicated**.[2] The vast majority of human diseases can be categorized as multifactorial, which are also referred to as complex diseases. They are caused by variation in many genes and they may or may not be influenced by the environment.

Trauma

Trauma or **traumatic** disease is caused by a physical injury from an external force. Trauma is the leading cause of death in children and young adults. The type of trauma or traumatic disease most commonly affecting individuals varies with age, race, and residence. For example, accidents, especially falls, are a common cause of traumatic disease in older adults, while gunshot wounds are the most common cause of traumatic disease and even death in young adult black males living in urban areas.[3] However, motor vehicle crashes are the most frequent cause of serious injury overall.

Inflammation

Inflammation is a complex reaction in tissues that consists mainly of responses of blood vessels and **leukocytes**. The body's principal defenders against foreign **invaders** are plasma proteins and circulating leukocytes, as well as tissue **phagocytes** that are derived from circulating cells. The presence of proteins and leukocytes in the blood gives them the ability to home to[4] any site where they may be needed. Because invaders such as **microbes** and **necrotic** cells are typically present in tissues, outside the circulation, it follows that[5] the circulating cells and proteins have to be rapidly recruited to these **extravascular** sites.

Inflammation may contribute to a variety of diseases that are not thought to be primarily due to abnormal host responses. For instance, **chronic** inflammation may play a role in **atherosclerosis**, type 2 diabetes, **degenerative** disorders, and cancer. In recognition of the widely-ranging harmful consequences of inflammation, the **lay** press has rather **melodramatically** referred to it as "the silent killer".

Infection

An **infectious** disease or **communicable** disease is caused by a biological agent such as a **virus**, **bacterium**, or **parasite**. Infectious diseases are the **invasion** of a **host** organism by a foreign **replicator**, generally **microorganisms**, often called microbes, which are invisible to the naked eye.[6] Microbes that cause illness are also known as **pathogens**. The most common pathogens are various bacteria and viruses, though a number of other microorganisms, including some kinds of **fungi** and **protozoa**, also cause diseases. An infectious disease is termed **contagious** if it is easily **transmitted** from one person to another. An organism that a microbe infects is known as the host for that microbe. In the human host, a microorganism causes disease by either **disrupting** a vital body process or **stimulating** the immune system to mount a defensive reaction. An immune response against a pathogen, which can include a high fever, inflammation, and other damaging symptoms, can be more **devastating** than the direct damage caused by the microbe.

Neoplasm

Neoplasms or **tumors** may be classified as **benign** or **malignant**. Generally speaking, benign tumors are not deadly because they have limited growth and are **encapsulated**, thus easily removed. Malignant tumors are just the opposite. These tumors are usually deadly since they grow uncontrollably, and invade their surrounding tissues with finger-like or "crab-like" **projections**. This characteristic makes **surgical removal** of cancer quite difficult. Another characteristic of malignant neoplasms is that they **metastasize**. **Metastatic** cancers move from a site of origin to another secondary site in the body. For example, lung cancer commonly metastasizes to the bone. Malignant means deadly or progressing to death. With this definition, it is understandable why the terms tumor, **malignancy**, and cancer bring fear to an individual.

Impaired Immunity

The immune system of the body is a specialized group of cells, tissues, and organs that are designed to defend the body against **pathogenic** attacks. Impaired immunity, which refers to any of various failures in the body's defense mechanisms against infectious organisms, occurs when some part of this system **malfunctions**. Disorders of immunity include immune deficiency diseases, such as AIDS, that arise because of a **diminution** of some aspect of the immune response. Other types of immune disorders, such as **allergies** and **autoimmune** disorders, are caused when the body develops an inappropriate response to a substance—either to a normally harmless foreign substance found in the environment, in the case of allergies, or to a component of the body, in the case of autoimmune diseases.[7] **Lymphocytes** can become cancerous and give rise to tumours called **leukemia**, **lymphoma**, and **myeloma**.

With advances in understanding the mechanisms of disease, it has become clear that the fundamental causes of diseases are mostly based on biochemical and biophysical responses within the cell. Although a disease may have one principal **etiologic** agent, it is becoming increasingly apparent that there are usually several factors involved in a disease process. Discovering a contributing factor and characterizing its contribution to a disease are a difficult **undertaking**, because the effect of any single factor may be **obscured** or **confounded** by other contributing factors. The ultimate goal of learning the mechanisms of disease is to identify these factors in the hope of successful **therapy** and disease prevention.

▶ **Word Bank**

trauma /'trɔ:mə/ *n.* 创伤，外伤

inflammation /ˌɪnflə'meɪʃən/ *n.* 发炎，炎症

neoplasm /'ni:əʊplæzəm/ *n.* 赘生物，肿瘤

impair /ɪm'peə/ *v.* 损害

immunity /ɪ'mju:nɪtɪ/ *n.* 免疫

chromosomal /ˌkrɒmə'səməl/ *a.* 染色体的

monogenic /ˌmɒnəʊ'dʒenɪk/ *a.* 单基因的

multifactorial /ˌmʌltɪfæk'tɔ:rɪəl/ *a.* 多因子的

segregate /'segrɪgɪt/ *v.* 分离，分隔

Mendelian /men'di:lɪən/ *a.* 孟德尔的

chromosome /'krəʊməsəʊm/ *n.* 染色体

genome /'dʒi:nəʊm/ *n.* 基因组，染色体组

duplicate /'du:plɪkeɪt/ *v.* 复制

traumatic /trɔ:'mætɪk/ *a.* 创伤的；外伤的

leukocyte /'lju:kəsaɪt/ *n.* 白细胞，白血球

invader /ɪn'veɪdə/ *n.* 入侵者

phagocyte /'fægəsaɪt/ *n.* 吞噬细胞

microbe /'maɪkrəʊb/ *n.* 微生物

necrotic /ne'krɒtɪk/ *a.* 坏死的

extravascular /ˌekstrə'væskjʊlə/ *a.* 血管外的

chronic /'krɒnɪk/ *a.* 慢性的

atherosclerosis /ˌæθərəʊsklɪə'rəʊsɪs/ *n.* 动脉硬化，动脉粥样硬化

degenerative /dɪ'dʒenərətɪv/ *a.* 退行性的

lay /leɪ/ *a.* 世俗的；外行的

melodramatically /ˌmelədrə'mætɪkəlɪ/ *ad.* 戏剧性地

infectious /ɪn'fekʃəs/ *a.* 传染的

communicable /kə'mju:nɪkəbl/ *a.* 可传染的

virus /'vaɪrəs/ *n.* 病毒

bacterium /bæk'tɪərɪəm/ *n.* 细菌（复数为 bacteria）

parasite /'pærəsaɪt/ *n.* 寄生虫

invasion /ɪn'veɪʒən/ *n.* 入侵

host /həʊst/ *n.* 宿主

replicator /'replɪkeɪtə/ *n.* 复制因子

microorganism /ˌmaɪkrəʊ'ɔ:gənɪzəm/ *n.* 微生物

pathogen /'pæθədʒən/ *n.* 病原体

fungus /'fʌndʒəs/ *n.* 真菌（复数为 fungi）

protozoan /ˌprəʊtə'zəʊən/ *n.* 原生动物（复数为 protozoa）

contagious /kən'teɪdʒəs/ *a.* 感染性的；接触传染的

transmit /'trænsmɪt/ *v.* 传输，传送

disrupt /dɪs'rʌpt/ *v.* 扰乱

stimulate /'stɪmjʊleɪt/ *v.* 刺激

devastate /'devəsteɪt/ *v.* 毁灭

tumor /'tju:mə/ *n.* 肿瘤

benign /bɪ'naɪn/ *a.* 良性的

malignant /mə'lɪgnənt/ *a.* 恶性的

encapsulate /en'kæpsəleɪt/ *v.* 封进内部；装入胶囊

projection /prə'dʒekʃən/ *n.* 突出物

surgical /'sɜ:dʒɪkəl/ *a.* 外科的；手术的

removal /rɪ'mu:vəl/ *n.* 消除

metastasize /mə'tæstəsaɪz/ *v.* 转移，迁徙

metastatic /ˌmetə'stætɪk/ *a.* 转移性的

malignancy /mə'lɪgnənsɪ/ *n.* 恶性（肿瘤等）

pathogenic /ˌpæθə'dʒenɪk/ *a.* 致病的

malfunction /mæl'fʌŋkʃən/ *v.* 故障；功能障碍

diminution /ˌdɪmɪ'nju:ʃən/ *n.* 减少

allergy /'ælədʒɪ/ *n.* 过敏

autoimmune /ˌɔ:təʊɪ'mju:n/ *a.* 自身免疫的

lymphocyte /'lɪmfəsaɪt/ *n.* 淋巴细胞

leukemia /lju:'ki:mɪə/ *n.* 白血病

lymphoma /lɪm'fəʊmə/ *n.* 淋巴瘤

myeloma /ˌmaɪə'ləʊmə/ *n.* 骨髓瘤

etiologic /ˌi:tɪə'lɒgɪk/ *a.* 病因学的

undertaking /ˌʌndə'teɪkɪŋ/ *n.* 任务；工作

obscure /əb'skjʊə/ *v.* 使含混；变得模糊

confound /kən'faʊnd/ *v.* 使困惑

therapy /'θerəpɪ/ *n.* 治疗，疗法

▶ Notes

1. 该句为简单句，句子主干为 Mechanisms of disease reveal the functional and structural changes，其中宾语 changes 被三个定语修饰：形容词 functional 和 structural，介词短语 in disease，介词短语 from the molecule level to the effects on the individual。

2. 该句为并列句，由三个简单句构成，句型为 ... , ... , or ... 。每个简单句的谓语部分均由 may be + 形容词或 may + 动词被动语态构成，形成平行关系。

3. 该句为并列句，连词 while 表示转折，强调两个分句的对比。在第一个分句中，介词短语 in older adults 作定语，修饰 traumatic disorders；在第二个分句中，介词短语 in young adult black males 作定语，修饰 traumatic disease and even death，现在分词短语 living in urban areas 作定语，修饰 young adult black males。

4. home to 意为定居于。home 此处为不及物动词，表示定居或安家，后面可跟 to、on 或 at，表示定居地点，例如：People who are in favor of living alone always home at the place far away from the downtown area.。

5. it follows that 意为由此得出结论。It follows that 常用于描述现象后引出观点，表示这一现象引起的结果或推导出的原理，可翻译为由此断定、由此可见或由此可知等，例如：He is wrong, but it does not follow that you are right.。

6. 该句为复合句，主句为 Infectious diseases are the invasion of a host organism by a foreign replicator，其中，a host organism 意为被入侵者，a foreign replicator 意为入侵者，过去分词短语 often called microbes 修饰 foreign replicator 的同位语 microorganisms，非限定性定语从句 which are invisible to the naked eye 修饰 microbes。

7. 该句为复合句，句子主干为 Other types of immune disorders are caused，在 when 引导的时间状语从句中，either ... or ... 分别连接两个平行结构 to a normally harmless foreign substance found in the environment, in the case of allergies 和 to a substance 和 to a component of the body, in the case of autoimmune diseases。

Exercises

Ⅰ. **Choose the best answer to each of the following questions.**

1. Scientists usually classify diseases into six categories based on _____.
    A. causes of the diseases
    B. effects of the diseases
    C. the rate of mortality
    D. structural changes of molecules

2. Diseases are divided into monogenic, chromosomal, or multifactorial, according to _____.
    A. the alteration in a single gene
    B. the genetic contribution
    C. the principles of inheritance
    D. the alteration of chromosomal makeup

3. Which group of people die from trauma more often than the other ones?
    A. Children and young adults.   B. Young adult black males.
    C. Older adults.   D. Middle-aged adults.

4. The main defenders of the body include plasma proteins, tissue phagocytes, and _____.
    A. circulating cells   B. foreign invaders
    C. circulating leukocytes   D. necrotic cells

5. Why is inflammation considered as "the silent killer" by the lay press?
    A. Because inflammation has various harmful effects on people.
    B. Because acute inflammation may turn into chronic inflammation.
    C. Because inflammation is the primary cause of many diseases.
    D. Because inflammation may cause diabetes, atherosclerosis, and even cancer.

6. An infectious disease is identified as contagious once _____.
    A. the body is invaded by microbes
    B. pathogens are discovered in the body
    C. a host organism does not function properly
    D. it is passed on easily from person to person

7. Benign tumors differ from malignant ones in that the former _____.
    A. usually progress rapidly   B. do not metastasize
    C. grow unlimitedly   D. grow uncontrollably

8. Removing cancer in surgery is quite difficult because _____.
    A. cancer usually metastasizes to bones
    B. cancer is most often dangerous
    C. cancer always moves to the secondary site
    D. cancer has finger-like projections to tissues nearby

9. When will our body have impaired immunity?
    A. When the body develops a response to a substance.
    B. When the immune system malfunctions.
    C. When the immune system defends us against pathogens.
    D. When lymphocytes become active.

10. Why is it difficult to discover a contributing factor of a disease?

    A. Because there are several factors involved in a disease.

    B. Because a disease has one principal etiologic agent.

    C. Because there are many biochemical responses in cells.

    D. Because the effect of a single factor may not be singled out.

Ⅱ. **Fill in each blank with a proper word mentioned in Text A. The first letter of the word is given.**

1. Eating d_____ are conditions defined as abnormal eating habits that may involve either insufficient or excessive food intake.

2. Redness, swelling, and fever are signs of i_____ when something harmful or irritating affects part of our body.

3. The physical injury to the body caused by an external source is also known as t_____.

4. Neoplasm is used as a synonym of t_____, which is caused by the abnormal growth or division of cells.

5. The key to avoiding poor blood c_____ is to find an optimal combination of exercise and diet to maintain your overall cardiovascular health.

6. COVID-19 is an i_____ disease caused by a newly discovered coronavirus.

7. In popular culture the term m_____ is often used to refer to microorganisms, although often in a negative context.

8. Lipoma（脂肪瘤）, which is not deadly, is the second most common b_____ tumor of the colon.

9. We used a combined regimen（治疗方案）of injection treatment and physical t_____ for the disease.

10. Acupuncture anesthesia is rapidly gaining ground in s_____ operations.

Ⅲ. **Fill in each blank in the following paragraph with a word in the box. Change the form of words if necessary.**

biochemical	symptom	specialize	disease	organic
clinical	systemic	syndrome	cause	pathological
broad	therapy	result	abnormal	technique

Pathology is the study of 1_____. More specifically, it is devoted to the study of the structural, 2_____, and functional changes in cells, tissues, and organs that underlie disease. By the use of molecular, microbiologic, immunologic, and morphologic 3_____, pathology attempts to explain the whys and wherefores (理由) of the signs and 4_____ manifested by patients while providing a rational basis for clinical care and 5_____. It thus serves as the bridge between the basic sciences and 6_____ medicine, and is the scientific foundation for all of medicine. Traditionally the study of pathology is divided into general pathology and 7_____ pathology. The former is concerned with the reactions of cells and tissues to 8_____ stimuli and to inherited defects, which are the main 9_____ of disease. The latter examines the alternations in 10_____ organs and tissues that are responsible for disorders that involve these organs.

IV. Translate the following English sentences into Chinese.

1. Mechanisms of disease reveal the functional and structural changes in disease from the molecular level to the effects on the individual.

2. Because invaders such as microbes and necrotic cells are typically present in tissues, outside the circulation, it follows that the circulating cells and proteins have to be rapidly recruited to these extravascular sites

3. In the human host, a microorganism causes disease by either disrupting a vital body process or stimulating the immune system to mount a defensive reaction.

4. These tumors are usually deadly since they grow uncontrollably, and invade their surrounding tissues with finger-like or "crab-like" projections.

5. Other types of immune disorders, such as allergies and autoimmune disorders, are caused when the body develops an inappropriate response to a substance—either to a normally harmless foreign substance found in the environment, in the case of allergies, or to a component of the body, in the case of autoimmune diseases.

V. Write a summary (120w–150w) of the mechanisms of disease.

Reading

Text B   Alzheimer's Disease and Treatment

When Alois Alzheimer first described the disease in 1906, a person in the United States lived an average of about 50 years. Few people reached the age of greatest risk. As a result, the disease was considered rare and attracted little scientific interest. That attitude changed as life span increased and scientists began to realize how often Alzheimer's disease (AD) strikes people in their 70s and 80s. The U.S. Department of Health and Human Services recently estimated the average life expectancy to be 79.6 years. Today AD is at the **forefront** of biomedical research.

AD is a **neurological** disorder in which the death of brain cells causes memory loss and cognitive decline. Like all types of **dementia**, it is a **neurodegenerative** disease, which means there is **progressive** brain cell death that happens over a course of time. The disease starts mild and gets progressively worse. The **incidence** of AD rises **exponentially** with advancing age. The total brain size shrinks with AD—the tissue has progressively fewer nerve cells and connections. Estimates vary, and according to the Alzheimer's Association in the U.S., AD affects around 5.5 million Americans, most of them over the age of 65, and is the sixth leading cause of death in the U.S.

The major **underlying** mechanism of AD is the accumulation of proteins called beta-**amyloid** and tau within the brain. Although we still do not know what starts the disease process, it can go on for many years without symptoms, which is called the **preclinical** or **presymptomatic** stage of the disease.[1] With the **progression** of AD, it can be broken down into three basic stages: mild, **moderate**, and severe stages.

As more and more beta-amyloid **plaques** and **neurofibrillary tangles** (**aggregates** of tau) form in particular brain areas, healthy neurons begin to work less efficiently, then lose their ability to function and communicate with each other, and eventually die. This process seems to begin in the parts of the brain responsible for forming new memories, in particular, the **hippocampus** and **entorhinal cortex**. The early **symptomatic** stage of AD is called mild cognitive impairment. At the time, the minor changes in the person's abilities or behavior are often mistakenly attributed to stress or **bereavement** or, in older people, to the normal process of aging. It is often only when looking back that we realize that these signs were probably the beginnings of dementia.

At the moderate stage, with the death of more neurons, affected brain regions begin to shrink, leading to functional problems, which are the signs and symptoms of AD. As AD progresses, plaques and tangles spread throughout the brain, starting in the **neocortex**.[2] Damage occurs in areas of the brain that control language, reasoning, **sensory** processing, and conscious thought. Memory loss and confusion increase, and people begin to have problems recognizing family members and friends. They may be unable to learn new things, carry out tasks that involve multiple steps (such as getting dressed) or cope with new situations. They may have **hallucinations**, **delusions**, and **paranoia** and may behave **impulsively**. Imaging of the brain often reveals **atrophy** of the **parietal** and **medial temporal lobes**.

By the final stage, plaques and tangles have spread throughout the brain, and brain tissue has shrunk significantly. People with severe AD cannot communicate and are completely dependent on others for their care. Near the end, the person may be in bed most or all of the time, as the body shuts down. Generalized **cerebral** atrophy with **posterior predominance** may be seen on imaging.

There are no drug treatments available that can provide a cure for AD. However, medicines have been developed that can improve symptoms, or temporarily slow down their progression, in some people. There are two main types of medication used to treat AD: **cholinesterase inhibitors** and **NMDA receptor antagonists**, which work in different ways.

Cholinesterase inhibitors include **donepezil hydrochloride** (Aricept), **rivastigmine** (Exelon), and **galantamine** (Reminyl). Between 40 and 70 percent of people with AD benefit from cholinesterase inhibitor treatment, but it is not effective for everyone and may improve symptoms only temporarily, between 6 and 12 months in most cases. According to an Alzheimer's Society survey of 4,000 people, those using these treatments often experience improvements in motivation, anxiety levels, and confidence, in addition to daily living, memory, and thinking.

NMDA receptor antagonist is **memantine** (Ebixa). Memantine is licensed for the treatment of moderate-to-severe AD. It can temporarily slow down the progression of symptoms, including everyday function, in people in the middle and later stages of the disease. There is evidence that memantine may also help behavioral symptoms such as aggression and **agitation**.

Although there is not necessarily a way to stop AD from developing, there are many things people can do to stay healthy as they age and thus decrease their environmental and lifestyle risks. These healthy habits include eating a nutritious diet, exercising regularly, staying socially engaged, participating in mentally stimulating activities, and maintaining a consistent sleep schedule.

The more we understand about this disease, the more complicated it appears to become. Fortunately, the high level of research activity offers hope for a brighter future of the care of AD patients. With the **advent** of[3] advances in molecular biology, genetics, **pharmacology**, and **biochemistry**, we have learned so much about the disease process that **mechanistic** approaches to both diagnosis and treatment now seem within reach⁴. The search for **biomarkers** of the disease has greatly advanced. Very soon it will be possible to take a blood test to make a diagnosis of AD. We are also closer to being able to image the **pathology** of AD in a living person's brain, enabling **clinicians** to accurately diagnose an individual at the earliest possible stage of dementia.

▶ Word Bank

forefront /'fɔːfrʌnt/ *n.* 前沿

dementia /dɪ'menʃə/ *n.* 痴呆

neurodegenerative /ˌnjuːrəudɪ'dʒenərətɪv/ *a.* 神经退行性的

progressive /prə'gresɪv/ *a.* 进行性的，渐进性的

exponentially /ˌekspəu'nenʃɪəlɪ/ *ad.* 以指数方式地

amyloid /'æmɪlɔɪd/ *n.* 淀粉样蛋白

presymptomatic /ˌprɪsɪmptə'mætɪk/ *a.* 症状发生前的

moderate /'mɒdərət/ *a.* 适度的，中等的

neurofibrillary /ˌnjuərə'faɪbrɪlərɪ/ *n.* 神经原纤维

aggregate /'ægrɪgɪt/ *n.* 聚合物

entorhinal /ˌentə'raɪnəl/ *a.* 内嗅的

symptomatic /ˌsɪmptə'mætɪk/ *a.* 有症状的；症状的

neocortex /ˌnɪəu'kɔːteks/ *n.* 新（大脑）皮质

hallucination /həˌluːsə'neɪʃən/ *n.* 幻觉

paranoia /ˌpærə'nɔɪə/ *n.* 偏执

atrophy /'ætrəfɪ/ *n.* 萎缩

medial /'miːdɪəl/ *a.* 中间的

lobe /ləub/ *n.* 脑叶

posterior /pəu'stɪərɪə/ *a.* 其次的；后部的

cholinesterase /ˌkəulɪ'nestəreɪz/ *n.* 胆碱酯酶

NMDA N- 甲基 -D- 天冬氨酸（N-methyl-D-aspartic acid 的缩写形式）

receptor /rɪ'septə/ *n.* 受体

donepezil /ˌdʌnə'piːzəl/ *n.* 多奈哌齐

rivastigmine /ˌraɪvəs'tɪgmɪn/ *n.* 卡巴拉汀

motivation /ˌməutɪ'veɪʃən/ *n.* 动机，积极性

agitation /ˌædʒɪ'teɪʃən/ *n.* 焦虑不安

pharmacology /ˌfɑːmə'kɒlədʒɪ/ *n.* 药物学，药理学

mechanistic /ˌmekə'nɪstɪk/ *a.* 机械论的，机械学的

pathology /pə'θɒlədʒɪ/ *n.* 病理学

neurological /ˌnjuərə'lɒdʒɪkəl/ *a.* 神经学的

incidence /'ɪnsɪdəns/ *n.* 发生率

underlying /ˌʌndə'laɪɪŋ/ *a.* 潜在的；根本的

preclinical /prɪ'klɪnɪkəl/ *a.* 临床前的

progression /prə'greʃən/ *n.* 进展

plaque /plæk/ *n.* 斑块

tangle /'tæŋgl/ *n.* 缠结

hippocampus /ˌhɪpə'kæmpəs/ *n.* 海马体

cortex /'kɔːteks/ *n.* 皮质，皮层

bereavement /bɪ'riːvmənt/ *n.* 丧失（尤指亲友）

sensory /'sensərɪ/ *a.* 感觉的；知觉器官的

delusion /dɪ'luːʒən/ *n.* 妄想，错觉

impulsively /ɪm'pʌlsɪvlɪ/ *ad.* 冲动地

parietal /pə'raɪɪtəl/ *a.* 颅顶骨的；腔壁的

temporal /'tempərəl/ *a.* 颞的，太阳穴的；时间的

cerebral /sə'riːbrəl/ *a.* 大脑的；脑的

predominance /prɪ'dɒmɪnəns/ *n.* 优势；显著

inhibitor /ɪn'hɪbɪtə/ *n.* 抑制剂

antagonist /æn'tægənɪst/ *n.* 拮抗剂

hydrochloride /ˌhaɪdrəu'klɔːraɪd/ *n.* 氢氯化物

galantamine /gə'læntəmɪn/ *n.* 加兰他敏

memantine /'meməntaɪn/ *n.* 美金刚胺，美金胺

advent /'ædvənt/ *n.* 到来，出现

biochemistry /ˌbaɪəu'kemɪstrɪ/ *n.* 生物化学

biomarker /ˌbaɪəu'mɑːkə/ *n.* 生物标记

clinician /klɪ'nɪʃən/ *n.* 临床医生

▶ Notes

1. 该句为复合句，主句为 it can go on for many years without symptoms，it 指代让步状语从句中的 the disease process。Although we still do not know what starts the disease process 为让步状语从句，其中包含了一个宾语从句 what starts the disease process。非限定性定语从句 which is called the preclinical or presymptomatic stage of the disease 修饰主句的内容，即 the disease process can go on for many years without symptoms。

2. 该句为复合句，主干为 affected brain regions begin to shrink，现在分词短语 leading to functional problems 为结果状语，非限定性定语从句 which are the signs and symptoms of AD 修饰 functional problems。

3. with the advent of 意为随着……的到来，尤其指不寻常的人或物的出现，例如：With the advent of managed care in the United States, the conversation over the direction of medicine has become laden with economic terms.。

4. within reach 意为指日可待，reach 在该介词短语中表示智力、影响、能力等所及范围，例如：They had been looking at condos（托管公寓），but the sharp drop in housing prices made bigger homes within reach.。

Exercises

Ⅰ. **For each of the following statements, write "T" if the statement is true and "F" if the statement is false in the blank.**

_____ 1. When AD was first described as a disease, the life span in America was only about 50 years.

_____ 2. AD is a unique type of dementia, which triggers the death of cells progressively.

_____ 3. Generally speaking, AD falls into three basic phases: mild, moderate, and severe.

_____ 4. At the mild stage, minor alterations in the person's behavior are often regarded as a result of normal aging.

_____ 5. With the progression of AD, plaques and tangles start spreading throughout the brain at the final stage.

_____ 6. At the moderate stage, along with an increase in brain size, signs and symptoms of AD occur.

_____ 7. AD is not an incurable disease, as many medicines have been developed for its treatment.

_____ 8. Cholinesterase inhibitors have some therapeutic effects on 40 to 70 percent of people with AD according to the passage.

_____ 9. Memantine can be used only for the treatment of moderate-stage AD.

_____ 10. Scientists will probably be able to diagnose AD with a blood test very soon.

Ⅱ. **Match each term in Column A with its corresponding description in Column B. Write the corresponding letter in the blank.**

Column A	Column B
_____ 1. dementia	A. the study of the chemical processes that occur in living things
_____ 2. impairment	B. a mental state characterized by a lack of clear thought
_____ 3. delusion	C. a small abnormal patch on or inside the body
_____ 4. inhibitor	D. a medical science that studies the causes and effects of diseases
_____ 5. clinician	E. a mental state of extreme emotional disturbance
_____ 6. pathology	F. a person who does clinical work instead of laboratory work
_____ 7. biochemistry	G. a substance that retards or stops an activity
_____ 8. plaque	H. the state of believing things that are not true
_____ 9. confusion	I. a symptom of reduced quality or strength
_____ 10. agitation	J. severe loss of intellectual capacity

Ⅲ. **Translate the following Chinese sentences into English.**

1. 阿尔茨海默病是脑细胞死亡导致记忆丧失和认知减退的一种神经性疾病。

2. 这个过程似乎从大脑负责形成新记忆的区域开始，尤其是海马体和内嗅皮层。

3. 大脑中支配语言、推理、感觉加工和意识思考的各区域会受到损伤。

4. 阿尔茨海默病协会对 4000 人的调查结果显示，接受这些药物治疗的患者不仅在日常生活、记忆力和思维能力上得到提高，而且其积极性、焦虑水平和自信心也得到改善。

5. 我们即将能够拍出阿尔茨海默病在活人脑中的病理影像，以帮助临床医生尽可能在人们出现痴呆的最早阶段作出准确诊断。

Ⅳ. **Think critically and then answer the following questions.**

1. Alzheimer's disease is the most common form of dementia, which worsens as it progresses and eventually leads to death. Although some medicines can temporarily slow down the progression of AD, unfortunately, there is no cure for this disease. Can you explain why it is so difficult to cure AD?

2. People usually fail to notice the symptoms of AD until the moderate stage when AD is very difficult to control, so it is important to examine the conditions in one's brain before the symptoms occur. As mentioned in the text, the accumulation of beta-amyloid and tau proteins is the mechanism behind AD. Do you think it is possible to develop a chemical test to make an early diagnosis of AD by detecting beta-amyloid and tau proteins?

Medicine in China

TCM's View of Disease

Traditional Chinese Medicine (TCM), a great treasure-house of culture, is an indispensable part of the splendid classic Chinese culture. In its long course of development, it has absorbed the quintessence of classical Chinese philosophy, culture and science, and summarized the experience of the Chinese people in fighting against disease. It is rich in theory and practical in treatment. Today, modern medicine is quite advanced, but TCM is still widely used because of its significant clinical curative effect.

TCM lays particular stress on the importance of harmony to health, holding that a person's physical health depends on harmony in the functions of the various body organs, the moderate status of the emotional expression, and adaption and compliance to different environments, of which the most vital is the dynamic balance between *yin* and *yang*. The fundamental cause of illness is that various internal and external factors disturb the dynamic balance. Therefore, maintaining health actually means conserving the dynamic balance of body functions, and curing diseases means restoring chaotic body functions to a state of coordination and harmony.

Exercises

Ⅰ. **Translate the underlined part into Chinese.**

Ⅱ. **Answer the following question.**

What is TCM's view of disease?

Chapter 4

Skeletal System

Pre-Reading Question

What is the meaning of "a skeleton in the closet"? Do you know somebody who has a skeleton in the cupboard?

Reading

Text A Structure and Functions of the Skeletal System

Bone formation begins early in **fetal** development when the **skeleton** is composed mostly of **cartilage** and continues to grow and develop until a person is 25 years old. The human skeleton consists of 300 bones at birth and by the time adulthood is reached, some bones have **fused** together to give a total of 206 bones in the body. The skeletal bone mass reaches its maximum **density** by age 30.

In addition to bones, the skeletal system includes **ligaments**, **tendons**, and joints. Movement is possible because bones provide points and attachment for ligaments, tendons, and muscles. The human skeleton serves some other functions. The most obvious function of the skeleton is to hold the body up. It also protects the inner organs and **passage-ways**. Bone tissues can store several minerals, including **calcium** and **phosphate**. When required, bone releases minerals into the blood and facilitates the balance of minerals in the body. Red blood cells are produced within the bone **marrow**. Bone cells release a hormone called **osteocalcin**, which increases the insulin **secretion** and sensitivity.

Despite appearing dry and lifeless, our bones are alive and active because they have blood vessels, nerves, and living bone cells known as **osteocytes**. These are held together by a framework of hard, non-living material containing calcium and phosphate. A thin membrane called the **periosteum** covers the surface of your bones. Running along the center of long bones, such as your **femur** (thigh bone), is a **medullary** cavity filled with bone marrow.[1] Red bone marrow is a soft tissue that produces blood cells and yellow bone marrow is a store for fat. Bone can either be

spongy or **compact**. Spongy bone is lightweight and made up of a **mesh** of needle-like pieces of bone with large spaces between them. Compact bone is dense and forms the outer layer of all your bones.

Adult bones come in several different shapes and sizes. The shape of a bone reflects its role within your body. Long bones, like in your arms and legs, are mostly made of compact bone. Short bones, like the ones in your wrists and ankles, are mainly made of spongy bone. Flat bones, like your rib and skull bones, are made of a layer of spongy bone sandwiched between two thin layers of compact bone. Irregular bones, such as your **pelvic girdle**, are oddly shaped bones that do not fit into the other three groups.

When two or more bones meet, a joint is formed. Every bone in the body—except for the **hyoid** bone in the throat—meets up with at least one other bone at a joint. A joint is also known as an **articulation**. The shape of a joint depends on its function. Joints hold your bones together and allow your rigid skeleton to move. Generally speaking, joints that allow a greater range of movement have a higher risk of injury. There are three types of joints. Immovable joints (**synarthroses**[2]), such as the **suture** joints of the skull, are fixed and do not allow any movement. Slightly movable joints (**amphiarthroses**) are capable of little movement. The **intervertebral discs** come under this category. Freely movable joints (**diarthroses** or **synovial** joints), such as the knee and elbow joints, are highly movable and help the body to move.

The human skeleton can be divided into two parts: the **axial** skeleton (80 bones) and the **appendicular** skeleton (126 bones) (Figure 4–1). The axial skeleton is formed by the vertebral column (26 vertebrae), the **thoracic** cage (12 pairs of ribs and the **sternum**[3]), and the skull (22 bones and 7 associated bones). The upright posture of humans is maintained by the axial skeleton, which transmits the weight from the head, the trunk, and the upper **extremities** down to the lower extremities at the hip joints. The bones of the **spine** are supported by many ligaments. The **erector spinae** muscles are also supporting and are useful for balance. The vertebral column consists of five sections of **vertebrae**[4]: **cervical**, thoracic, **lumbar**, **sacral**, and **coccygeal** vertebrae. Cervical vertebrae connect the vertebral column and the **cranium**. The **sacrum** and **coccyx** at the base of the spine are formed by the **fusion** of **rudimentary** bones and thus are often called "sacral bone" or "coccygeal bone" as a unit. The sacrum makes up the junction between the vertebral column and the pelvic bones and is not considered as part of the axial skeleton. The purpose of the thoracic cage is to offer protection of the internal organs from injury while the main function of the cranium is to protect the brain and the organs of sight and hearing.

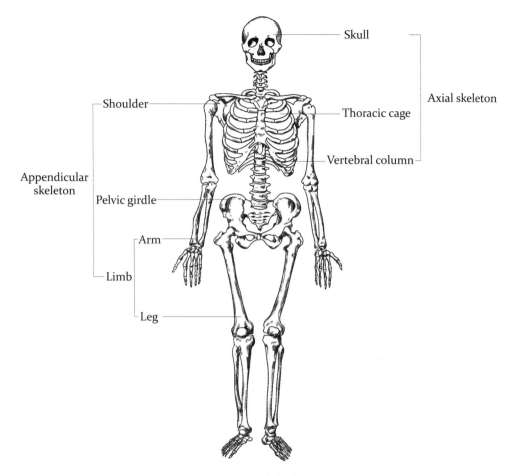

Figure 4-1   Structure of the human skeleton

The appendicular skeleton, which is attached to the axial skeleton, consists of the bones of **appendages** (upper limbs and lower limbs or arms and legs), along with the shoulder and pelvic girdles. The upper (**anterior**) limbs are attached to the top of the rib cage by the **pectoral** (shoulder) girdle and the lower (posterior) limbs are attached to the lower part of the spinal column by the pelvic (hip) girdle. Together, all the bones of the appendicular skeleton function to make **locomotion** possible and to protect the major organs of digestion, **excretion**, and **reproduction**.

The human skeletal system is equally important, when compared with other body systems. It gives our body a definite shape and structure and protects the vital organs. It can be called the basic **infrastructure** of our body, without which the human body would have been a ball-like structure rolling on the floor.[5]

▶ **Word Bank**

fetal /'fi:təl/ *a.* 胎的，胎儿的

cartilage /'kɑ:tɪlɪdʒ/ *n.* 软骨

density/'densɪtɪ/ *n.* 密度

tendon /'tendən/ *n.* 腱

calcium /'kælsɪəm/ *n.* 钙

marrow /'mærəʊ/ *n.* 髓，骨髓

secretion /sɪ'kri:ʃən/ *n.* 分泌；分泌物

periosteum /ˌperɪ'ɒstɪəm/ *n.* 骨膜，管膜

medullary /'medəˌlərɪ/ *a.* 骨髓的，髓质的；脊髓的

compact /'kɒmpækt/ *a.* 紧密的

pelvic /'pelvɪk/ *a.* 骨盆的

hyoid /'haɪɒɪd/ *a.* 舌骨的

synarthrosis /ˌsɪnɑ:'θrəʊsɪs/ *n.* 不动关节（复数为 synarthroses）

suture /'su:tʃə/ *n.* 缝合，缝合处

amphiarthrosis /ˌæmfɪɑ:'θrəʊsɪs/ *n.* 微动关节，丛和关节（复数为 amphiarthroses）

intervertebral /ˌɪntə'vɜ:tɪbrəl/ *a.* 椎间的

diarthrosis /ˌdaɪɑ:'θrəʊsɪs/ *n.* 动关节（复数为 diarthroses）

synovial /sɪ'nəʊvɪəl/ *a.* 滑液的；分泌滑液的

appendicular /ˌæpən'dɪkjʊlə/ *a.* 阑尾的；附属物的；四肢的

thoracic /θɔ:'ræsɪk/ *a.* 胸的，胸廓的

extremity /ɪks'tremɪtɪ/ *n.* 四肢；骨端；末端

erector spinae /ɪ'rektə 'spaɪni:/ *n.* 骶棘肌，竖脊肌

vertebra /'vɜ:tɪbrə/ *n.* 椎骨，脊椎（复数为 vertebrae）

lumbar /'lʌmbə/ *a.* 腰的，腰部的

coccygeal /kɒk'sɪdʒɪəl/ *a.* 尾骨的

sacrum /'seɪkrəm/ *n.* 骶骨

fusion /'fju:ʒən/ *n.* 融合

appendage /ə'pendɪdʒ/ *n.* 附件

pectoral /'pektərəl/ *a.* 胸的，胸部的

excretion /ɪk'skri:ʃən/ *n.* 排泄；排泄物；分泌；分泌物

reproduction /ˌri:prə'dʌkʃən/ *n.* 繁殖，生殖

skeleton /'skelɪtən/ *n.* 骨架，骨骼

fuse /fju:z/ *v.* 融合

ligament /'lɪgəmənt/ *n.* 韧带

passage-way /'pæsɪdʒweɪ/ *n.* 通道，通路

phosphate /'fɒsfeɪt/ *n.* 磷酸盐

osteocalcin /ˌɒstɪə'kælsɪn/ *n.* 骨钙蛋白

osteocyte /'ɒstɪəʊsaɪt/ *n.* 骨细胞

femur /'fi:mə/ *n.* 股骨，大腿骨

spongy /'spʌndʒɪ/ *a.* 海绵状的；多孔而有弹性的

mesh /meʃ/ *n.* 网眼

girdle /'gɜ:dl/ *n.* 围绕物

articulation /ɑ:ˌtɪkjʊ'leɪʃən/ *n.* 关节

disc /dɪsk/ *n.* 圆盘

axial /'æksɪəl/ *a.* 轴的，轴向的

sternum /'stɜ:nəm/ *n.* 胸骨

spine /spɒɪn/ *n.* 脊柱，脊椎

cervical /'sɜ:vɪkəl/ *a.* 颈的；子宫颈的

sacral /'seɪkrəl/ *a.* 骶骨的

cranium /'kreɪnɪəm/ *n.* 颅骨，头盖骨

coccyx /'kɒksɪks/ *n.* 尾骨，尾椎

rudimentary /ˌru:dɪ'mentərɪ/ *a.* 初步的，未发展的

anterior /æn'tɪərɪə/ *a.* 前面的；先前的

locomotion /ˌləʊkə'məʊʃən/ *n.* 运动，移动

infrastructure /'ɪnfrəstrʌktʃə/ *n.* 下部构造

▶ Notes

1. 该句是倒装句，将表语部分 running along the center of long bones, such as your femur (thigh bone) 置于主语 a medullary cavity filled with bone marrow 之前，主要目的是强调和突出表语。本句正常语序应为：A medullary cavity filled with bone marrow is running along the center of long bones, such as your femur (thigh bone)。

2. synarthroses 源于希腊语，是 synarthrosis 的复数。希腊语以 "-is" 结尾的名词变复数时，将 -is 变成 -es。如：amphiarthroses（微动关节）是 amphiarthrosis 的复数，diarthroses（动关节）是 diarthrosis 的复数，diagnoses（诊断）是 diagnosis 的复数，paralyses（麻痹）是 paralysis 的复数，dermatoses（皮肤病）是 dermatosis 的复数。

3. sternum 的复数为 sterna，源于拉丁语。拉丁语中以 "-um" 结尾的名词变复数时将 um 变成 a。如：ovum（卵子）的复数为 ova，cranium 的复数为 crania，sacrum 的复数为 sacra。许多拉丁语名词都被英语同化，因此有些拉丁语名词有两个复数形式，一个是英语的，另一个是拉丁语的。上面的几个单词的复数也可以是 sternums、ovums、craniums 及 sacrums。

4. vertebrae 是 vertebra 的复数，源于拉丁语。拉丁语中以 "-a" 结尾的名词变复数时在词尾加 e，如：amoeba（阿米巴）的复数是 amoebae。

5. 该定语从句使用了虚拟语气，表示对过去事件的纯粹假设，因而谓语部分由 would 加完成式构成。without which the human body would have been a ball-like structure rolling on the floor 是修饰 infrastructure 的非限定性定语从句，在定语从句中先行词 infrastructure 作介词 without 的宾语。

Exercises

Ⅰ. **Choose the best answer to each of the following questions.**

1. What comprises the skeletal system?
   A. All the muscles, ligaments, and tendons in the body.
   B. All the bones and the cells produced by the bone marrow.
   C. All the organs, including both soft and hard tissue organs.
   D. All the bones in the body and the tissues that connect them.

2. Which function of the skeletal system would be especially important if you had a car accident?
   A. Storage of minerals.　　　　　B. Protection of inner organs.
   C. Facilitation of movement.　　　D. Fat storage.

3. The hollow space in the middle of bones is filled with _____.
   A. air　　　　　　　　　　　B. blood
   C. bone marrow　　　　　　　D. bone cells

4. What works with the bones of your skeleton to make your body move?
   A. Diarthroses.　　　　　　　B. Muscles.
   C. Cartilages.　　　　　　　　D. Organs.

5. The vertebrae belong to _____.
   A. the axial skeleton   B. the appendicular skeleton
   C. the thoracic cage   D. the synarthroses

6. What are the bones found in the cranium?
   A. Short bones.   B. Long bones.
   C. Regular bones.   D. Flat bones.

7. Blood cells are formed in _____.
   A. the osteocytes   B. the red bone marrow
   C. the periosteum   D. the compact bone

8. The thoracic bones provide protection for _____.
   A. the heart and lungs   B. the brain
   C. the pelvic organs   D. the hearing organs

9. What does the cranium protect in addition to the brain?
   A. The osteocytes.   B. The sense organs.
   C. The diaphragm.   D. The heart.

10. A good example of a synovial joint is _____.
    A. the vertebra   B. the cranial suture joint
    C. the elbow joint   D. the intervertebral disc

Ⅱ. **Write the types (long bone, short bone, flat bone, irregular bone) of the bones in the spaces given.**

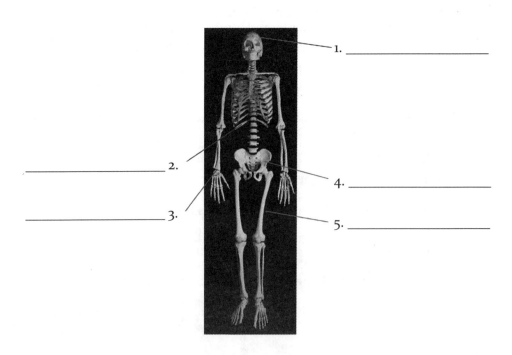

1. _____

2. _____

3. _____

4. _____

5. _____

Ⅲ. Fill in each blank in the following paragraph with a word in the box. Change the form of words if necessary.

medullary	spongy	rest	vessel	constant
tissue	skeleton	marrow	high	bone
remain	impact	convert	compact	circulation

Bones are strong and hard. Bones have a hard outer layer called the 1_____ bone. This outer layer makes up about 80% of the total bone mass of an adult 2_____ . The inside of the bone is called the cancellous (多孔的) or 3_____ bone. The cancellous tissue makes up the 4_____ 20% of the total bone mass and provides space for blood 5_____ and marrow. The bone marrow is found in the 6_____ cavities of most major bones. Not only does red bone marrow produce blood cells to maintain 7_____ blood levels, but it also helps to remove old cells from 8_____ . Yellow 9_____ consists primarily of fat cells. When blood supply is extremely low, it can be 10_____ to red marrow in order to produce more blood cells.

Ⅳ. Translate the following English sentences into Chinese.

1. Bone formation begins early in fetal development when the skeleton is composed mostly of cartilage and continues to grow and develop until a person is 25 years old.

2. When required, bone releases minerals into the blood and facilitates the balance of minerals in the body.

3. The upright posture of humans is maintained by the axial skeleton, which transmits the weight from the head, the trunk, and the upper extremities down to the lower extremities at the hip joints.

4. The purpose of the thoracic cage is to offer protection of the internal organs from injury.

5. The human skeletal system can be called the basic infrastructure of our body, without which the human body would have been a ball-like structure rolling on the floor.

Ⅴ. Write a 100-word summary of the classification and function of joints.

Reading

Text B   Diseases of the Skeletal System and Their Treatment

Skeletal disorders include pathologic conditions associated with bone, cartilage, ligaments, and joints.

Bone Fractures

The most common traumatic injury to a bone is a fracture, or break. When this occurs, there is swelling due to injury and bleeding tissues. The common types of fractures are **greenstick**, closed/simple, open/compound, and **comminuted**. Greenstick is the simplest type of fracture. The bone is partly bent, but it never completely separates. Such fractures are common among children because their bones contain flexible cartilage. In closed/simple fracture, the bone is broken, but the broken ends do not pierce through the skin to form an external wound. An open/compound is considered to be a most serious type of fracture, where the broken bone ends pierce and **protrude** through the skin. This can cause infection of the bone and its neighboring tissues. A fracture is comminuted when the bone is broken into many pieces that can become **embedded** in the surrounding tissues.[1]

Treatment of the fracture consists of reduction[2] or **realignment** of the broken bones. This may be accomplished through the use of **traction** or may include the use of surgically placed rods, plates, and/or screws. **Immobilization** of the bone during the healing process is achieved with a **cast** or **splint**.

Bone Infection

Osteomyelitis is an inflammation or infection of the bone caused by bacteria entering a wound or carried by the blood into the bone.[3] It most commonly occurs in children between the ages of 5 and 14 years. Intense **antibiotic** treatment is usually required to **eradicate** an infection.

Metabolic Bone Diseases

Osteoporosis is a disorder in which bones lose minerals and become less dense, leading to an increased risk of fracture. Osteoporosis is most common in women after the **menopause**, when it is called **postmenopausal** osteoporosis, but may develop in men and **premenopausal** women in the presence of[4] particular hormonal disorders and other chronic diseases or as a result of smoking and medications, specifically **glucocorticoids**. Treatment or preventive measures may include medication, weight-bearing exercise, and a good source of calcium and vitamin D.

Rickets and **osteomalacia** (softening of the bone) occur due to a deficit of vitamin D and the resultant lack of calcium absorption. Rickets is more often seen in children who have soft bones due to lack of **calcification**, causing such **deformities** as **bowlegs** and pigeon breast. The disease may be prevented with sufficient quantities of calcium, vitamin D, and exposure to sunshine. Osteomalacia is seen in adults who have poor vitamin D absorption as well, resulting in **compression** fractures of the vertebrae.

Tumors of Bone

Osteosarcoma, or bone cancer, is the most common and devastating malignant neoplasm of bone. The most common sites of **infliction** are the **distal** femur and **proximal** areas of the **tibia** and **humerus**. Nearly twice as many males as females are affected and most cases occur between 20 and 40 years of age. Osteosarcoma is characterized by severe, **unrelenting** pain. Treatment involves surgical removal of the tumor and both presurgical and postsurgical **chemotherapy**. **Chondrosarcoma** is a tumor that arises from the cartilage and is more often seen in adults. Treatment is surgical removal of the lesion and chemotherapy is not effective in treating chondrosarcoma.

Joint Disorders

Joint disorders can be classified as **noninflammatory** or inflammatory joint diseases. Traumatic injury is often the cause of noninflammatory joint problems. A **dislocation** occurs when a bone is displaced from its proper position in a joint. This may result in the tearing and stretching of the ligaments. Reduction or return of the bone to its proper position is necessary, along with rest to allow the ligaments to heal. A **sprain** is an injury to a joint caused by any sudden or unusual motion. The ligaments are either torn from their attachments to the bones or torn across, but the joint is not dislocated. A sprain is accompanied by rapid swelling and acute pain in the area and is treated with nonsteroid **anti-inflammatory** drugs.

Osteoarthritis, known as degenerative joint disease, is the most common noninflammatory disorder of movable joints. As one ages, the **articular** cartilage degenerates and bony **spur** formation occurs at the joint. The joints may enlarge; there is pain and swelling, especially after activity.

Arthritis is a general term for many different inflammatory joint diseases. It can be caused by a variety of factors, including infection, injury, genetic factors, and **autoimmunity**. **Rheumatoid** arthritis is a chronic, autoimmune disease which affects the connective tissue and joints. There is acute inflammation of the connective tissue, thickening of the synovial membrane, and **ankylosis** (fused joints). The joints are badly swollen and painful. This disease affects approximately three times more women than men. At present, there is no cure for arthritis although there are many treatments including medications to reduce pain and inflammation, rest, and/or physical therapy. If fluid accumulates in the joint, an **arthrocentesis** may be necessary to drain the fluid and relieve the pressure in the joint.

Abnormal Curvatures of the Spine

Kyphosis (hunchback) is a **humped** curvature in the thoracic area of the spine. **Lordosis** is an exaggerated inward curvature in the lumbar region of the spine just above the sacrum. **Scoliosis** is a side-to-side or lateral curvature of the spine.

A disc that protrudes into the spinal canal and puts pressure on the spinal nerve is called a **herniated** disc. It can be diagnosed with a CT scan (noninvasive test using computed **tomography**), MRI, or a **myelogram**. Medications are used to reduce the inflammation and decrease pain and muscle **spasms**. Rest is often encouraged along with strengthening exercises, depending on the extent of the herniation.

▶ Word Bank

fracture /'fræktʃə/ *n.* 骨折

comminuted /'kɒmɪnjuːtɪd/ *a.* 粉碎性的

embed /ɪm'bed/ *v.* 嵌入

traction /'trækʃən/ *n.* 牵引

cast /kɑːst/ *n.* 石膏

osteomyelitis /ˌɒstɪəʊˌmaɪə'laɪtɪs/ *n.* 骨髓炎

eradicate /ɪ'rædɪkeɪt/ *v.* 消除

menopause /'menəpɔːz/ *n.* 绝经；更年期

premenopausal /ˌpriːmɪnə'pɔːzəl/ *a.* 绝经前的

rickets /'rɪkɪts/ *n.* 佝偻病

calcification /ˌkælsɪfɪ'keɪʃən/ *n.* 钙化

bowleg /'bəʊleg/ *n.* 内弯腿

osteosarcoma /ˌɒstɪəʊsɑː'kəʊmə/ *n.* 骨肉瘤

distal /'dɪstəl/ *a.* 远端的，末端的

tibia /'tɪbɪə/ *n.* 胫骨

unrelenting /ˌʌnrɪ'lentɪŋ/ *a.* 无情的；不松懈的

chemotherapy /ˌkiːməʊ'θerəpɪ/ *n.* 化疗

chondrosarcoma /ˌkɒndrəʊsɑː'kəʊmə/ *n.* 软骨肉瘤

noninflammatory /nɒnˌɪn'flæmətərɪ/ *a.* 非炎性的

dislocation /ˌdɪsləʊ'keɪʃən/ *n.* 关节脱位

anti-inflammatory /ˌæntaɪɪn'flæmətərɪ/ *a.* 抗炎的；消炎的

greenstick /'griːnstɪk/ *n.* 青枝骨折

protrude /prə'truːd/ *v.* 突出

realignment /ˌriːə'laɪnmənt/ *n.* 重新排列，重新定线

immobilization /ɪˌməʊbəlaɪ'zeɪʃən/ *n.* 固定

splint /splɪnt/ *n.* 夹板

antibiotic /ˌæntɪbaɪ'ɒtɪk/ *a.* 抗菌的；抗生素

osteoporosis /ˌɒstɪəʊpə'rəʊsɪs/ *n.* 骨质疏松症

postmenopausal /ˌpəʊstmenəʊ'pɔːzəl/ *a.* 绝经后的

glucocorticoid /ˌgluːkəʊ'kɔːtɪkɔɪd/ *n.* 糖皮质激素

osteomalacia /ˌɒstɪəʊmə'leɪʃə/ *n.* 软骨病

deformity /dɪ'fɔːmətɪ/ *n.* 畸形

compression /kəm'preʃən/ *n.* 压迫；压缩；浓缩

infliction /ɪn'flɪkʃən/ *n.* 侵害

proximal /'prɒksɪməl/ *a.* 近端的

humerus /'hjuːmərəs/ *n.* 肱骨

sprain /spreɪn/ *n.* 扭伤

osteoarthritis /ˌɒstɪəʊɑːˈθraɪtɪs/ *n.* 骨关节炎

articular /ɑːˈtɪkjʊlə/ *a.* 关节的

spur /spɜː/ *n.* 刺

arthritis /ɑːˈθraɪtɪs/ *n.* 关节炎

autoimmunity /ˌɔːtəʊɪˈmjuːnɪtɪ/ *n.* 自身免疫

rheumatoid /ˈruːmətɔɪd/ *a.* 类风湿性的

ankylosis /ˌæŋkɪˈləʊsɪs/ *n.* 关节僵硬

arthrocentesis /ˌɑːθrəʊsenˈtiːsɪs/ *n.* 关节穿刺（术）

curvature /ˈkɜːvətʃə/ *n.* 弯曲

kyphosis /kaɪˈfəʊsɪs/ *n.* 驼背

hunchback /ˈhʌntʃbæk/ *n.* 驼背

humped /hʌmpt/ *a.* 隆起的

lordosis /lɔːˈdəʊsɪs/ *n.* 脊柱前弯症

scoliosis /ˌskəʊlɪˈəʊsɪs/ *n.* 脊柱侧凸

herniate /ˈhɜːnɪeɪt/ *v.* 疝出

tomography /təˈmɒɡrəfɪ/ *n.* 断层扫描术

myelogram /ˈmaɪələʊˌɡræm/ *n.* 脊髓 X 光像

spasm /ˈspæzəm/ *n.* 痉挛，抽搐

▶ Notes

1. 该句中 when 引导时间状语从句，that 引导定语从句，修饰 many pieces。become/be embedded in something 这个短语的意思为嵌入到……中。

2. reduction 一词在该句中不是减少的意思。在医学英语中，reduction 指复位，即将骨头恢复到合适的位置。

3. 该句中现在分词短语 entering a wound 和过去分词短语 carried by the blood into the bone 都作定语修饰名词 bacteria。

4. in the presence of… 是介词短语，在该句中作条件状语，表示"患有……"，也可表示"存在有……"或"在……的情况下"。

Exercises

Ⅰ. **For each of the following statements, write "T" if the statement is true and "F" if the statement is false in the blank.**

_____ 1. In the case of a simple fracture, the skin at the site is damaged.

_____ 2. The bacterial inflammation of the bone marrow is known as osteoporosis.

_____ 3. Vitamin D deficiency can lead to osteomalacia in adults.

_____ 4. Chondrosarcoma is a malignant bone cancer that strikes adults more often.

_____ 5. Rheumatoid arthritis may ultimately lead to systemic inflammation.

_____ 6. Kyphosis is a humped curvature in the thoracic region of the spine.

_____ 7. The cause of arthritis is not known.

_____ 8. Osteosarcoma often inflicts the proximal areas of the tibia and humerus.

_____ 9. In osteoporosis, bones lose minerals and have decreased density.

_____ 10. Dislocation should be treated with nonsteroid anti-inflammatory drugs.

Ⅱ. **Match each term in Column A with its correct description in Column B. Write the corresponding letter in the blank.**

Column A	Column B
_____ 1. osteomalacia	A. an inflammatory joint disease
_____ 2. closed fracture	B. degeneration of articular cartilage
_____ 3. osteomyelitis	C. abnormal side-to-side curvature of the spine
_____ 4. arthritis	D. bacterial infection of the bone marrow
_____ 5. arthrocentesis	E. cancer of the cartilage
_____ 6. osteoarthritis	F. joint injury caused by sudden motion
_____ 7. scoliosis	G. bone broken, skin intact
_____ 8. myelogram	H. softening of the bone
_____ 9. sprain	I. an X-ray image of the spinal column
_____ 10. chondrosarcoma	J. a procedure to remove fluid from a joint

Ⅲ. **Translate the following Chinese sentences into English.**

1. 当骨头断裂为许多碎块并嵌入周围组织时即为粉碎性骨折。

2. 愈合过程中采用石膏或夹板来固定骨头。

3. 男性和绝经前的女性如果患有某种激素失调症和其他慢性疾病，或者由于吸烟和使用某些药物，也会患骨质疏松症。

4. 随着年龄的增长，关节软骨退化，关节中形成骨刺。

5. 脊柱前弯症是骶骨上方的腰椎部分向内过度弯曲。

Ⅳ. **Think critically and then answer the following questions.**

1. Two patients were admitted to the emergency room yesterday. The first

case was a 15-year-old boy who had a tibia and fibula (腓骨) fracture. The second case was a 36-year-old woman whose knee articular cartilage had been damaged. Which of the two patients would recover faster? And why?

2. Mr. Wang experienced severe sharp pain in his lower back while lifting heavy boxes. The pain was not relieved by traditional home remedies or painkillers. He finally went to see a doctor after 48 hours. What was wrong with him? And what diagnosis would the doctor make?

Medicine in China

Bionic Bones Strengthen the Future of Orthopedic Implants

Chinese researchers are designing bionic bones with improved biological compatibility and mechanical strength, which will bring new possibilities for future orthopedic implants.

Researchers from Northwestern Polytechnical University have spent more than 15 years developing artificial bones that are highly consistent with the composition, structure, and mechanical properties of natural bones.

Wang Yan'en from the university, which is based in Xi'an, Shaanxi Province, led his team in experimenting with hundreds of different solutions to create a binder that would not only result in a strong and robust scaffold but also adapt to the biological environment. The researchers used hydroxyapatite, a medical bioceramic material, to fabricate bone scaffolds. Wang said that although it is considered as one of the most suitable materials for bone scaffold fabrication, bonding the powderlike material into a strong and robust scaffold remains difficult.

Wang's team also explored how to use 3D printing technology to make customized bone scaffolds. They cooperated with companies in developing 3D bionic bone printing machines.

Exercises

Ⅰ. **Translate the underlined part into Chinese.**

Ⅱ. **Answer the following question.**

What significance do the bionic bones designed by Chinese researchers have?

Chapter 5

Muscular System ◀

Pre-Reading Question

What does "flex your muscles" mean? Can you list some examples of "flex one's muscles"?

Reading

Text A Structure and Functions of the Muscular System

Muscle, an essential tissue of the human body, provides force for various movements of the body. Without the muscles to fill in those spaces in the skeletal system, imagine how a human body would look like.[1]

The muscular system consists of 639 muscles that can flex, contract, and stretch to perform a variety of body movements. Muscle is made up of muscle **fibers** which are elongated cells containing **contractile** elements that are responsible for[2] changing the size and shape of muscle so that it produces a force of movement. Hence, it is a contractile tissue and is primarily designed for movements. Action of various muscles may result in either movements of various parts of the body and the body as a whole or movements of internal organs of the body.

These movements can be **voluntary** and **involuntary**. The voluntary movements are those that you can control consciously, while the involuntary are movements that you cannot control. Muscle contractions cause these body movements and occur when **actin** and **myosin filaments** slide over each other.

Interestingly, the word "muscle" is derived from the Latin word "**musculus**" which means mouse. Certain muscles resemble a mouse with their tendon representing the mouse tail.

The muscular system can be broken down into three types of muscles: skeletal, smooth, and cardiac (Figure 5–1), based on their locations in relation to various body parts and on their functions.

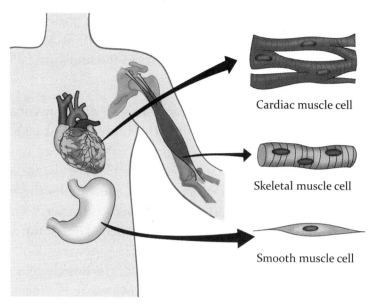

Cardiac muscle cell

Skeletal muscle cell

Smooth muscle cell

Figure 5-1   Three types of muscles

Skeletal muscles are probably the most abundant type of muscle because **virtually** all these muscles are attached to the bones of the skeletal system. They are the muscles that ache after **strenuous** work or exercise and collectively constitute about 40 percent of the body's mass or weight. Skeletal muscles are attached to bones by tough, **fibrous** connective tissues called tendons. Tendons are rich in protein collagen, which is arranged in a **wavy** way so that they can stretch and provide additional length at the muscle-bone junction.

Skeletal muscles are considered as a form of **striated** muscles that are set into operation and controlled by the **somatic** nervous system. In other words, skeletal muscles are subjected to movement or resist against a move with an individual's own will, and that is why you can call them voluntary contractile organs. Concerning their location, as the very name suggests[3], these muscles are associated with the bony skeleton and are firmly attached to the bones through collagen fibers or tendons.

Skeletal muscles act in pairs. The **flexing** (contracting) of one muscle is balanced by the lengthening (relaxation) of its paired muscle or a group of muscles. These **antagonistic** (opposite) muscles can open and close joints such as the elbow or knee. Examples of antagonistic muscles are the **biceps** and the **triceps**[4]. When the biceps muscle flexes, the **forearm** bends in at the **elbow** toward the biceps; at the same time, the triceps muscle lengthens. When the forearm is bent back out in a straight-arm position, the biceps lengthens and the triceps flexes.

Muscles that contract and cause a joint to close, such as the biceps, are called

flexor muscles. Those that contract and cause a joint to open, such as the triceps, are called **extensors**. Skeletal muscles that support the skull, backbone, and rib cage are called axial skeletal muscles. Skeletal muscles of the limbs are called distal skeletal muscles.

Exclusively found in the heart, cardiac muscle (also called **myocardium**) is responsible for pumping blood throughout the body. The heart's natural **pacemaker** is made of cardiac muscle that signals other cardiac muscles to contract. Like skeletal muscles, the cardiac or heart muscles are also striated, but unlike the former, the latter are involuntary and do not come under the voluntary control of an individual. The cardiac muscle cells contract in coordination with the cells in close **proximity**[5] and as a result, the blood is propelled out of the **atria** and **ventricles**. These vital heart muscles are ensured ample supply of blood through the **coronary** arteries. By means of this circulatory fluid, the muscle cells not only get **replenished** with oxygen but are also able to remove waste products, such as carbon dioxide.

As opposed to the other two major types of muscles, smooth muscles are not only involuntary in action but also non-striated in appearance. In terms of their location, the smooth muscle tissues are scattered across many parts of the body, such as blood vessels (including arteries and veins), **lymphatic** vessels, **uterus**, urinary bladder, respiratory tract, male and female reproductive tracts, gastrointestinal tract, the **ciliary** muscles, **iris** of the eye, and **arrector pili** of the skin. The smooth muscle cells located in different organs of the body show structural and functional similarities, but there is a **substantial** difference in the nature of inducing stimuli. This significant **disparity** in inducing stimuli is very necessary so that individually desired effects are performed in the body at individual time. The contraction of a smooth muscle is caused by its **excitation** which is, in turn, induced by external stimuli. When the filaments of actin and myosin slide across each other, the result is the contraction of smooth muscles. Contraction is followed by relaxation, thus **initiating** a **rhythmic** impulse across the length of the vessel or tract.

Apart from producing movements, muscle performs other important functions for the body: **rendering** stability, maintaining posture, and generating heat. The desirable strength and stability for your **erect** standing posture are rendered by the support and efficiency of muscles. The balance of the body is ensured by your brain with the help of muscles, and if there were no such contractile organs, you would never be able to either stand or sit but would keep on lying on the ground or just make **sluggish** and **staggering** movements. Muscles help to maintain posture through a continual partial contraction of skeletal muscles. This process is known as **tonicity**. Besides, muscles generate heat as they contract. This heat is vitally important in maintaining normal body temperature.

Although not usually cited as a major muscle function, skeletal muscles also protect fragile internal organs by **enclosure**. What's more, smooth muscle, in particular, forms **valves** to regulate the passage of substances through internal body openings.

▶ Word Bank

fiber /'faɪbə/ *n.* 纤维

voluntary /'vɒlən,tərɪ/ *a.* 随意的

actin /'æktɪn/ *n.* 肌动蛋白

filament /'fɪləmənt/ *n.* 肌丝；细丝

virtually /'vɜːtjʊəlɪ/ *ad.* 事实上；几乎

fibrous /'faɪbrəs/ *a.* 纤维的；纤维性的

striated /straɪ'eɪtɪd/ *a.* 纹状的

flex /'fleks/ *v.* 屈曲，弯曲

biceps /'baɪseps/ *n.* 二头肌

forearm /'fɔːrɑːm/ *n.* 前臂

flexor /'fleksə/ *n.* 屈肌

myocardium /,maɪəʊ'kɑːdɪəm / *n.* 心肌

proximity /prɒk'sɪmətɪ/ *n.* 接近，邻近

ventricle /'ventrɪkl/ *n.* 心室；脑室

replenish /rɪ'plenɪʃ/ *v.* 补充

uterus /'juːtərəs/ *n.* 子宫

iris /'aɪrɪs/ *n.* 虹膜

pilus /'paɪləs/ *n.* 毛，发（复数为 pili）

disparity /dɪ'spærətɪ/ *n.* 不同，差异

initiate /ɪ'nɪʃɪeɪt/ *v.* 开始，发起

render /'rendə/ *v.* 致使

sluggish /'slʌgɪʃ/ *a.* 行动迟缓的

tonicity /təʊ'nɪsɪtɪ/ *n.* 紧张性，张力

valve /vælv/ *n.* 瓣，瓣膜；阀

contractile /kən'træktəl/ *a.* 收缩的

involuntary /ɪn'vɒlən,tərɪ/ *a.* 不随意的；非自愿的

myosin /'maɪəsɪn/ *n.* 肌球蛋白

musculus /'mʌskjʊləs/ *n.* 肌，肌肉

strenuous /'strenjʊəs/ *a.* 紧张的；费力的；艰苦的

wavy /'weɪvɪ/ *a.* 波状的，起伏的

somatic /səʊ'mætɪk/ *a.* 躯体的；体壁的

antagonistic /æn,tægə'nɪstɪk/ *a.* 拮抗的，对抗的，相克的

triceps /'traɪseps/ *n.* 三头肌

elbow /'elbəʊ/ *n.* 肘部

extensor /ɪk'stensə/ *n.* 伸肌

pacemaker /'peɪsmeɪkə/ *n.* 起搏点，起搏器

atrium /'eɪtrɪəm/ *n.* 心房（复数为 atria）

coronary /'kɒrənərɪ/ *a.* 冠状的；冠状动脉的

lymphatic /lɪm'fætɪk/ *a.* 淋巴的

ciliary /'sɪlɪərɪ/ *a.* 睫状的；睫的

arrector /ə'rektə/ *n.* 立肌

substantial /səb'stænʃəl/ *a.* 大量的；实质的

excitation /,eksaɪ'teɪʃən/ *n.* 激发，刺激

rhythmic /'rɪðmɪk/ *a.* 有节律的

erect /ɪ'rekt/ *a.* 竖立的，直立的

stagger /'stægə/ *v.* 蹒跚

enclosure /ɪn'kləʊʒə/ *n.* 附件；围墙

▶ Notes

1.　该句属于较为含蓄的虚拟语气，without sth/sb, 主语 + would 表示与现在或将来的事实相反的假设。

2.　与通用英语的词汇不同，医学英语词汇通常不具有感情色彩。例如，在普通英语中，be responsible for 通常译为对……负责，而在医学英语中，则译为引起、发挥……作用，不具有任何感情色彩。

3. as the very name suggests 可译为顾名思义。这里 very 表强调，用来加强语气，无实际意义，翻译成中文时常省略。

4. biceps 和 triceps 分别指二头肌和三头肌，bi-（二）和 tri-（三）是拉丁语中表示数量的前缀，例如：biangulate（有两角的），bicarbonate（重碳酸盐），triacid（三价酸），triglyceride（甘油三酯）等。

5. in close proximity 为介词短语，意思是邻近的，非常接近的，在本句中作定语，修饰 cells。

Exercises

Ⅰ. **Choose the best answer to each of the following questions.**

1. How does muscle produce movement?
   A. Through the change of muscle size and shape.
   B. Through contractile elements in muscle fibers.
   C. Through the interaction of internal organs.
   D. Through the support of the skeletal system.

2. What is the most abundant substance found in tendons?
   A. Actin filaments.   B. Myosin filaments.
   C. Protein collagen.   D. Muscle fibers.

3. Why are skeletal muscles called voluntary contractile organs?
   A. Because they are striated muscles.
   B. Because they are associated with skeletons.
   C. Because they can contract by themselves.
   D. Because they are controlled by an individual's own will.

4. The action between biceps and the triceps is _____.
   A. mutual   B. inhibitory
   C. antagonistic   D. cooperative

5. What can be said about the biceps?
   A. It can only flex, but not lengthen.
   B. It can only lengthen, but not flex.
   C. It is a type of axial skeletal muscle.
   D. It is a type of flexor muscle.

6. Cardiac muscles differ a lot from skeletal muscles mainly because _____.
   A. cardiac muscles are not striated

B. cardiac muscles are exclusively found in the heart

C. cardiac muscles are involuntary

D. cardiac muscles comprise the heart's natural pacemaker

7. The significant difference between various smooth muscle cells is marked by their _____.

A. structure   B. function

C. nature of stimulus induction   D. location

8. What causes the contraction of smooth muscles?

A. Excitation.

B. Involuntary action.

C. Filaments of actin and myosin.

D. Non-striated appearance.

9. With the help of muscles, the balance of the body is achieved by _____.

A. internal organs   B. external stimuli

C. our brain   D. body strength

10. According to the passage, valves are formed by _____.

A. smooth muscles   B. cardiac muscles

C. skeletal muscles   D. tendons

Ⅱ. **Match each term in Column A with its corresponding description in Column B. Write the corresponding letter in the blank.**

Column A	Column B
_____ 1. collagen	A. the muscular tissue of the heart
_____ 2. biceps	B. a fibrous protein
_____ 3. flexor	C. a muscle that stretches a body part
_____ 4. myocardium	D. the state of tissue tone or tension
_____ 5. filament	E. a very fine thread or threadlike structure
_____ 6. antagonistic	F. the large muscle in the back of the upper limb
_____ 7. extensor	G. a two-headed muscle in the upper limb
_____ 8. triceps	H. circular diaphragm forming the colored portion of the eye
_____ 9. iris	I. acting in opposition
_____ 10. tonicity	J. muscle that contracts and causes a joint to close

Ⅲ. Fill in each blank in the following paragraph with a word in the box. Change the form of words if necessary.

dilation	strength	tissue	posture	organ
extension	involuntarily	impulse	ligament	familiar
limb	visible	skeleton	voluntarily	position

Skeletal muscles are the muscles that cover the human skeleton. They are the muscles that are 1 _____ to us and can be felt. They help in holding up the bones of the human 2 _____ together and maintaining a proper 3 _____ of the body. Skeletal muscles are the most popular muscles and you must be familiar with them. The contraction and 4 _____ of skeletal muscles can be controlled 5 _____, indicating that when we think of contracting them, our nervous system transmits a(n) 6 _____ to do so. These muscles are connected to the bones, tendons, and 7 _____. They help in the movement of the 8 _____, enabling us to perform functions of walking, sitting, jumping and running. They also provide 9 _____ and support to the body and protect the internal 10 _____.

Ⅳ. Translate the following English sentences into Chinese.

1. Muscle is made up of muscle fibers which are elongated cells containing contractile elements that are responsible for changing the size and shape of muscle so that it produces a force of movement.

2. Skeletal muscles are probably the most abundant type of muscle because virtually all these muscles are attached to the bones of the skeletal system.

3. Exclusively found in the heart, cardiac muscle (also called myocardium), is responsible for pumping blood throughout the body.

4. As opposed to the other two major types of muscles, smooth muscles are not only involuntary in action but also non-striated in appearance.

5. Apart from producing movement, muscle performs other important functions for the body: rendering stability, maintaining posture, and generating heat.

Ⅴ. Write a 100-word summary of the characteristics and functions of biceps and triceps.

Reading

Text B　Diseases of the Muscular System and Their Treatment

A number of painful and troublesome medical conditions have been found to be associated with your muscular system. Some are easily curable, while others are chronic and may last for longer durations, and some are even incurable if not identified and addressed earlier. Depending upon[1] the type and seriousness of the situation, the patient may consult or get the help of **orthopedists**, **rheumatologists**, and **neurologists**. In most of the cases, the patient suffers from acute, severe or chronic pain or discomfort in the muscles, joints, and the surrounding areas.

Muscular **dystrophy** is a group of muscle diseases that weaken the **musculoskeletal** system and **hamper** locomotion. Muscular dystrophies are characterized by progressive skeletal muscle weakness, defects in muscle proteins, and the death of muscle cells and tissues. The diagnosis of muscular dystrophy is based on the results of muscle **biopsy**, increased serum **creatine phosphokinase**, **electromyography**, **electrocardiography**, and DNA analysis. There is no specific treatment for any form of muscular dystrophy. **Physiotherapy**, aerobic exercise, low-intensity **anabolic steroids**, and **prednisone** supplements may help to prevent **contractures** and maintain muscle **tone**. **Orthoses** and corrective **orthopedic** surgery may be needed to improve the quality of life in some cases. The **myotonia** (delayed relaxation of a muscle after a strong contraction) occurring in myotonic muscular dystrophy may be treated with medications such as **quinine**, **phenytoin**, or **mexiletine**, but no actual long-term treatment has been found.

Myasthenia gravis is a chronic autoimmune **neuromuscular** disease characterized by varying degrees of **episodic** weakness of the skeletal muscles of the body. The disorder is typically **mediated** by antibodies against the **postsynaptic acetylcholine** receptor or by antibodies against muscle-specific **tyrosine kinase**. The **hallmark** of myasthenia gravis is muscle weakness that increases during periods of activity and improves after periods of rest. Certain muscles such as those that control eye and eyelid movements, facial expression, chewing, talking, and swallowing are often, but not always, involved in the disorder. The muscles that control breathing and neck and limb movements may also be affected. Myasthenia gravis is caused by a defect in the transmission of nerve impulses to muscles. It occurs when normal communication between the nerve and muscle is interrupted at the neuromuscular junction—the place where nerve cells connect with the muscles they control. Myasthenia gravis is treated medically[2] with **acetylcholinesterase** inhibitors or **immunosuppressants**. The incidence of the disease is 3–30 cases per million per year and is rising as a result of increased awareness. Myasthenia gravis must be distinguished from **congenital myasthenic** syndromes that can present similar symptoms but do not respond to[3] **immunosuppressive** treatments.

Fibromyalgia is characterized by chronic widespread pain and **allodynia**. Its exact cause is unknown but is believed to involve psychological, genetic, neurobiological, and environmental factors. Symptoms of fibromyalgia are not just restricted to pain; **debilitating** fatigue, sleep disturbance, and joint stiffness are also clinically **manifested**. Some patients also report difficulty in swallowing, **bowel** and bladder abnormalities, numbness and **tingling**, and cognitive dysfunction. Fibromyalgia is frequently **comorbid**[4] with **psychiatric** conditions such as depression, anxiety, and stress-related disorders such as post-traumatic stress disorder. The administration of over-the-counter[5] painkillers, regular physical exercise, and psychological counseling may prove to be very beneficial for relieving the troubling symptoms of this disease. Although in some cases it becomes very difficult to **mitigate** the pains by any means, the abnormality is never life-threatening and does not bring about progressive disability or damages of the body.

Inflammatory muscle disease is an autoimmune disorder of unknown cause (**idiopathic**) which results in muscle weakness. The muscles involved are the muscles of the limbs, making movement difficult. Sometimes the muscles of swallowing or **phonation**, or even breathing may be involved. Rarely, facial muscles have weakness, as opposed to myasthenia gravis which frequently involves muscles of the eyes and face. In inflammatory muscle disease, the cardiac muscle may be involved, resulting in cardiac failure or **arrhythmias**. Sometimes, **myositis** may occur without other **manifestations** of disease, or myositis may be a part of a more **full-blown** autoimmune disorder, such as **systemic lupus erythematosus**. One of the standards of treatment for myositis is **corticosteroids**. Corticosteroids are powerful anti-inflammatory and **immunomodulatory** medications, and most cases of myositis will respond to corticosteroids alone. Sometimes, steroids are not enough by themselves, and the addition of "disease-modifying" drugs is necessary, for example, **methotrexate, azathioprine**, or even **cyclophosphamide**. A newer treatment option is to use **intravenous gamma globulin** for **refractory** cases. Sometimes, combinations of medications are necessary.

Muscle spasms and **cramps** are spontaneous and often painful muscle contractions. Cramps are usually defined as spasms that last over a period of time. Any muscle in the body may be affected, but spasms and cramps are most common in the **calves**, feet, and hands. While painful, spasms and cramps are harmless and are not related to any disorder, in most cases. Spasms or cramps may be caused by abnormal activities at any stage in the muscle contraction process, from the brain sending an electrical signal to the muscle fiber relaxing. Prolonged exercise, where sensations of pain and fatigue are often ignored, can lead to such severe energy shortages which make a muscle unable to relax, causing a spasm or cramp. **Dehydration**—the loss of fluids and salts through sweating, **vomiting**, or diarrhea—can disrupt **ion** balances in both muscles and nerves. This can prevent them from responding and recovering normally, which can result in spasms and cramps. Most simple spasms and cramps require no treatment other than[6] patience and stretching. Gentle stretching and massaging of the affected muscle may ease the pain and hasten recovery.

A **strain** is an injury to a muscle or tendon in which the muscle fibers tear as a result of overstretching. A strain is also **colloquially** known as a pulled muscle. The equivalent injury to a ligament is a sprain. Typical symptoms of a strain consist of localized stiffness, **discoloration** and **bruising** around the strained muscle. They can happen while doing everyday tasks and are not restricted to athletes. Nevertheless, people who play sports are more at risk of developing a strain due to increased muscle activities. Strains can be prevented by stretching and warming up before exercising and using proper lifting techniques.

▶ **Word Bank**

orthopedist /ˌɔːθəʊˈpiːdɪst/ *n.* 骨科医生，整形外科医师

neurologist /njʊəˈrɒlədʒɪst/ *n.* 神经病学家

musculoskeletal /ˌmʌskjʊləʊˈskelɪtəl/ *a.* 肌（与）骨骼的

hamper /ˈhæmpə/ *v.* 妨碍，束缚

creatine /ˈkriːətɪn/ *n.* 肌酸，甲胍基乙酸

electromyography /ɪˌlektrəʊmaɪˈɒɡrəfɪ/ *n.* 肌电描记法

electrocardiography /ɪˌlektrəʊˌkɑːdɪˈɒɡrəfɪ/ *n.* 心电描记法

physiotherapy /ˌfɪzɪəʊˈθerəpɪ/ *n.* 物理疗法

steroid /ˈstɪərɔɪd/ *n.* 类固醇，甾体

prednisone /ˈprednɪsəʊn/ *n.* 强的松（肾上腺皮质激素）

contracture /kənˈtræktʃə/ *n.* 挛缩

orthosis /ˈɔːθəʊsɪs/ *n.* 矫正法（复数为 orthoses）

orthopedic /ˌɔːθəʊˈpiːdɪk/ *a.* 整形外科的

quinine /ˈkwaɪnaɪn/ *n.* 奎宁

mexiletine /ˈmeksɪˌliːtiːn/ *n.* 美西律

myasthenia gravis /ˌmaɪæsˈθiːnɪə ˈɡrævɪs/ 重症肌无力

neuromuscular /ˌnjʊərəʊˈmʌskjʊlə/ *a.* 神经肌肉的

episodic /ˌepɪˈsɒdɪk/ *a.* 偶然发生的；短促的

postsynaptic /ˌpəʊstsɪˈnæptɪk/ *a.* 突触后的

tyrosine /ˈtaɪrəsiːn/ *n.* 酪氨酸

hallmark /ˈhɔːlmɑːk/ *n.* 特征，标志

rheumatologist /ˌruːməˈtɒlədʒɪst/ *n.* 风湿病学家

dystrophy /ˈdɪstrəfɪ/ *n.* 营养障碍，营养不良

biopsy /ˈbaɪɒpsɪ/ *n.* 活组织检查，活检

phosphokinase /ˈfɒsfəʊˌkɪneɪs/ *n.* 磷酸激酶

anabolic /ˌænəˈbɒlɪk/ *a.* 合成代谢的

tone /təʊn/ *n.* 紧张性

myotonia /ˌmaɪəʊˈtəʊnɪə/ *n.* 肌强直

phenytoin /ˈfenɪtɔɪn/ *n.* 苯妥英

mediate /ˈmiːdɪeɪt/ *v.* 调解；介导

acetylcholine /ˌæsetɪlˈkəʊliːn/ *n.* 乙酰胆碱

kinase /ˈkaɪneɪs/ *n.* 激酶

acetylcholinesterase /ˌæsetɪlkəʊlɪˈnestəreɪs/ n. 乙酰胆碱酯酶

immunosuppressant /ˌɪmjʊnəʊsəˈpresənt/ n. 免疫抑制剂

congenital /kənˈdʒenɪtəl/ a. 先天的，天生的 　　myasthenic /ˌmaɪəsˈθenɪk/ a. 肌无力的，肌衰弱的

immunosuppressive /ɪˈmjuːnəʊsəˈpresɪv/ a. 免疫抑制的

fibromyalgia /ˌfaɪbrəʊmaɪˈældʒɪə/ n. 纤维肌痛 　　allodynia /ˌæləʊˈdɪnɪə/ n. 异常性疼痛

debilitate /dɪˈbɪlɪteɪt/ v. 使衰弱 　　manifest /ˈmænɪfest/ v. 证明，表明，显示

bowel /ˈbaʊəl/ n. 肠 　　tingling /ˈtɪŋglɪŋ/ n. 麻刺感

comorbid /ˈkəʊmɔːbɪd/ v. 共病，（病症）同时存在 　　psychiatric /ˌsaɪkɪˈætrɪk/ a. 精神病学的

mitigate /ˈmɪtɪgeɪt/ v.（使）缓和，（使）减轻 　　idiopathic /ˌɪdɪəˈpæθɪk/ a. 特发的；先天的

phonation /fəʊˈneɪʃən/ n. 发声，发音 　　arrhythmia /əˈrɪθmɪə/ n. 心律不齐，节律失调

myositis /ˌmaɪəʊˈsaɪtɪs/ n. 肌炎

manifestation /ˌmænəfeˈsteɪʃən/ n.（临床）表现；显示；证明

full-blown /fʊlˈbləʊn/ a. 成熟的，充分发展的；严重的（疾病）

systemic /sɪˈstemɪk/ a. 系统的，全身的 　　lupus /ˈluːpəs/ n. 狼疮

erythematosus /ˌerɪθiːməˈtəʊsəs/ n. 红斑狼疮

corticosteroid /ˌkɔːtɪkəʊˈstɪrɔɪd/ n. 皮质激素，皮质类固醇；a. 皮质类固醇的

immunomodulatory /ˌɪmjʊnəʊˈmɒdjʊleɪtərɪ/ a. 免疫调节的

methotrexate /ˌmeθəˈtrekseɪt/ n. 甲氨蝶呤 　　azathioprine /ˌeɪzəˈθaɪəʊpriːn/ n. 咪唑硫嘌呤

cyclophosphamide /ˌsaɪkləʊˈfɒsfəmaɪd/ n. 环磷酰胺 　　intravenous /ˌɪntrəˈviːnəs/ a. 静脉内的

gamma /ˈgɑːmə/ n. γ（希腊语的第三个字母） 　　globulin /ˈglɒbjʊlɪn/ n. 球蛋白

refractory /rɪˈfræktərɪ/ a. 难治的 　　cramp /kræmp/ n. 痉挛，绞痛

calf /kɑːf/ n. 小腿，腓 　　dehydration /ˌdiːhaɪˈdreɪʃən/ n. 脱水

vomit /ˈvɒmɪt/ v. 呕吐 　　ion /ˈaɪən/ n. 离子

strain /streɪn/ n. 肌肉拉伤 　　colloquially /kəˈləʊkwɪəlɪ/ ad. 口语地

discoloration /dɪsˌkʌləˈreɪʃən/ n. 变色 　　bruising /ˈbruːzɪŋ/ n. 挫伤，瘀伤

▶ Notes

1. depending upon 意为根据，依靠，是现在分词形式用作状语，相当于 according to，又如：The amount of urine varies, depending on the fluids and foods a person consumes.（人排出的尿量不尽相同，这取决于其消耗的食物和水）。

2. medically 在此处表示在药物治疗方面。类似的副词还有 surgically 和 clinically 等，例如：Pituitary tumors can be removed surgically using the trans-sphenoidal approach, or their size can be reduced with irradiation.（垂体瘤可通过经蝶骨的方式用外科的方法摘除，或用放射法使其缩小）。

3. respond to 在该句中表示（药物）有效，因（药物）起作用而变好。

4. comorbid 一词由前缀 co-（意为合作、共同）和单词 morbid（意为病的、疾病的）构成。因此，comorbid 指的是病症同时存在。

5. over-the-counter 属于复合形容词，可缩写为 OTC，指的是非处方药。

6. no + 名词 + other than 表示除……外没有、只有、正是，又如：Many headaches are of short duration and require no treatment other than mild analgesics and rest.（很多头痛都是短期的，除少量服用一些镇痛剂及休息外，无须其他治疗）。

Exercises

Ⅰ. **For each of the following statements, write "T" if the statement is true and "F" if the statement is false in the blank.**

　　_____ 1. Muscular dystrophies are characterized by acute skeletal muscle weakness and defects in muscle proteins.

　　_____ 2. There is no specific treatment for any form of muscular dystrophy.

　　_____ 3. Myasthenia gravis is caused by a defect in the transmission of nerve impulses to the brain.

　　_____ 4. The typical feature of myasthenia gravis is muscle weakness that increases during activity and improves after taking medicine.

　　_____ 5. Congenital myasthenic syndromes can be treated with immunosuppressive medicines.

　　_____ 6. It is believed that fibromyalgia might be caused by psychological, genetic, neurobiological, and environmental factors.

　　_____ 7. If untreated, fibromyalgia would bring about life-threatening effects and progressive disability.

　　_____ 8. Facial muscles are often involved with weakness in inflammatory muscle disease.

　　_____ 9. In most cases, spasms and cramps are risk-free and are not associated with any disorder.

　　_____ 10. A strain is an injury to a muscle or ligament in which the muscle fibers tear as a result of overstretching.

Ⅱ. **Fill in each blank with a proper word mentioned in the text. The first letter of the word is given.**

　　1. A physician who corrects congenital or functional abnormalities of the bones with surgery is an o_____.

2. The act or power of moving from place to place is l_____.

3. The frequency with which something, such as a disease or trait, appears in a particular population or area is i_____.

4. Prolonged failure of muscle relaxation after contraction is called m_____.

5. Powerful medicines that inhibit the activity of the body's immune system are i_____.

6. A condition that damages or limits a person's physical or mental abilities is a d_____.

7. A general term for inflammation of the muscles is m_____.

8. A condition that occurs when the body loses more water than it takes in is d_____.

9. A muscle's painful long-lasting involuntary contractions are c_____.

10. An overstretching-induced injury to a ligamentis is a s_____.

Ⅲ. **Translate the following Chinese sentences into English.**

1. 重症肌无力是一种慢性自身免疫性神经肌肉疾病，以不同程度的发作性肌无力为特征。

2. 重症肌无力需与先天性肌无力综合征区分开，后者的症状与重症肌无力相似，但免疫抑制剂的治疗对其无效。

3. 纤维肌痛常与某些精神疾病共同发病，例如抑郁、焦虑及应激相关疾病（如创伤后应激障碍）。

4. 与经常累及眼外肌与面部肌的重症肌无力不同，炎性肌病极少对面部肌肉造成影响。

5. 从大脑发出电信号到肌纤维舒张，在肌肉收缩过程的任何阶段出现的异常活动都可能导致肌肉痉挛。

Ⅳ. **Think critically and then answer the following questions.**

1. The physician received a 3-year-old male child and then made the following synopsis of the visit: The mother states that she noticed her son has been falling a lot and seems to be very clumsy. She says that he has a wadding gait, is very slow in running and climbing, and walks on his toes. What might be the problem for the child? And what would be the corresponding intervention?

2.   Mr. Li was admitted to the hospital with a chief complaint of a condition marked by symmetrical weakness and pain. It was often accompanied by rashes around his eyes, face, and limbs. What diagnosis would the doctor make? And what treatment should be given to him?

Medicine in China

How Can Chinese Medicine Treat Myasthenia Gravis?

Chinese medicine may not be able to cure myasthenia gravis (MG), a chronic progressive disease characterized by chronic fatigue and muscular weakness (especially in the face and neck), but it can greatly help to manage and improve the symptoms of the disease.

Chinese medicine can also help improve the wellbeing and quality of life of MG patients and prevent the worsening and recurrence of the disease. After successful completion of the prescribed treatment plan, patients can resume a normal, symptom-free life. The Chinese medicine treatment includes Chinese herbal medicine, acupuncture, oriental dietary, and lifestyle advice. Exercise recommendations including Tai-chi, Qigong, or yoga will benefit MG patients massively.

Exercises

Ⅰ. **Translate the underlined part into Chinese.**

Ⅱ. **Answer the following question.**

How can Chinese medicine treat myasthenia gravis?

Chapter 6

Digestive System ◀

Pre-Reading Question

What is meant by the expression "down in the mouth"? Can you think of some similar expressions?

Reading

Text A Structure and Functions of the Digestive System

The digestive system (Figure 6–1) is uniquely constructed to perform its specialized function of turning food into energy and packaging the **residue** for waste **disposal**. It has two **anatomical subdivisions**, the digestive tract and the **accessory** organs. The digestive tract is a muscular tube extending from the mouth to the **anus**. It is also known as the **alimentary** canal that includes the **mouth, pharynx, esophagus**, stomach, and intestines. The stomach and intestines constitute the gastrointestinal tract. The accessory organs are the teeth, tongue, **salivary** glands, liver, **gallbladder**, and pancreas.

The first structure that food encounters on its way through the digestive system is the mouth, which is also the **uppermost** portion of the digestive tract where food is chewed and **moistened** to **facilitate** swallowing. After being chewed, food does not remain for long in the mouth; it is quickly swallowed and passes through the pharynx and down the esophagus to the stomach, where it is temporarily stored.

Just beyond the mouth, at the beginning of the tube leading to the stomach, is the pharynx.[1] Simply put[2], the pharynx is a common passageway for both respiration and digestion. The esophagus is a muscular tube that passes from the pharynx through the thoracic cavity and **diaphragm** into the abdominal cavity. By means of a series of muscular contractions called **peristalsis**, the esophagus delivers food to the stomach.

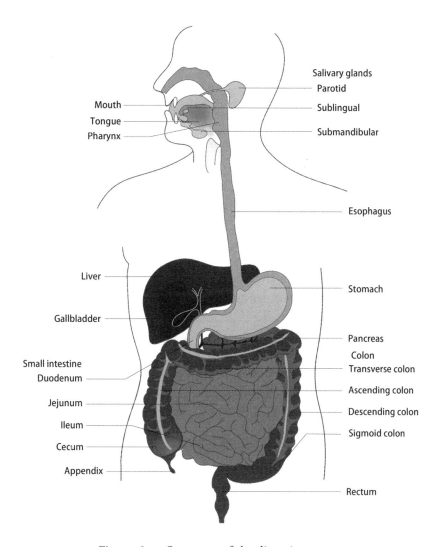

Mouth
Tongue
Pharynx

Salivary glands
Parotid
Sublingual
Submandibular

Esophagus

Liver
Gallbladder
Small intestine
Duodenum
Jejunum
Ileum
Cecum
Appendix

Stomach

Pancreas
Colon
Transverse colon
Ascending colon
Descending colon
Sigmoid colon

Rectum

Figure 6-1   Structure of the digestive system

The stomach is a thick-walled, J-shaped organ that lies on the left side of the abdominal cavity deep to the liver and diaphragm. Cells in the lining[3] of the stomach secrete strong acids and powerful enzymes that are responsible for the breakdown process. The length of the stomach remains at about 25 cm regardless of the amount of food it holds, but the **diameter** varies, depending on how full it is. There are four regions in the stomach. The cardiac region, which is in close proximity to the heart, surrounds the lower esophageal **sphincter** where food enters the stomach. The **fundic** region, which holds food temporarily, is an expanded portion superior to the cardiac region. The body region, which comes next, is the main part. The **pyloric** region narrows to become the pyloric canal leading to the pyloric sphincter through which food enters the **duodenum**, the first part of the small intestine.

The small intestine is found in the central and lower portions of the abdominal cavity, where it is supported by a fan-shaped **mesentery**. Made up of three segments—the duodenum, **jejunum**, and **ileum**—the small intestine breaks down food using enzymes released by the pancreas and **bile** from the liver. Peristalsis is also at work in this organ, moving food through and mixing it with digestive secretions from the pancreas and the liver. The duodenum is largely in charge of the continuous breaking-down process, with the jejunum and ileum mainly responsible for the absorption of nutrients into the bloodstream. Contents of the small intestine start out semi-solid and end in a liquid form after passing through the organ. Water, bile, enzymes, and **mucus** contribute to the change in consistency. Once the nutrients have been absorbed and the **leftover**—food residue liquid—has passed through the small intestine, it then moves on to the large intestine, or **colon**.

The large intestine begins in the lower right **quadrant** of the **peritoneal** cavity. It may be divided into the **cecum**, the colon, the **rectum**, and the **anal** canal. The cecum is a **pouch**-like structure forming the beginning of the large intestine. It is approximately three inches long with a small projection called the **vermiform appendix** as the attachment. The colon makes up the **bulk** of the large intestine and is segregated into several parts—the **ascending** colon, the **transverse** colon, the **descending** colon, and, at its end, the **sigmoid** colon. Digestion and absorption continue in the large intestine on a reduced scale. The waste products of digestion are eliminated from the body via the rectum and anus.

The **salivary** glands, pancreas, liver, and gallbladder are accessory organs of digestion. Ducts transport pancreatic juices from the pancreas and bile from the liver and gallbladder to the duodenum. The small intestine helps regulate the release of these juices by secreting hormones.

Resting on the posterior abdominal wall, the pancreas lies deep in the peritoneal cavity. It is an elongated and somewhat **flattened** organ that has both an endocrine function and an **exocrine** function.

The most **versatile** organ in the body is the liver, which is also the largest gland in the body and situated high in the abdomen on the right side—often reaching the fourth **intercostal** space, under the diaphragm. The liver plays an essential role in the normal metabolism of **carbohydrates**, fats, and proteins. In carbohydrate metabolism, it turns glucose into **glycogen** and stores it until needed by body cells. In some ways, the liver acts as the gatekeeper to the blood. As blood from the intestines passes through the liver, the liver removes poisonous substances and works to keep the contents of the blood constant. Additionally, it produces body heat and **detoxifies**[4] many potentially harmful substances such as drugs and alcohol.

The gallbladder is a pear-shaped muscular **sac** attached to the **ventral** surface of the liver. The liver produces bile, which enters many bile ducts associated with hepatic **lobules**[5]. These bile ducts join to form the common bile duct that enters the duodenum. Any excess bile backs up through the cystic duct into the gallbladder, where it is stored. Bile, which contains salts, bile **pigments**, **cholesterol**, and **electrolytes**, becomes **concentrated** in the gallbladder as water is absorbed.

▶ Word Bank

residue /'rezɪdjuː/ *n.* 残渣，剩余

anatomical /ˌænə'tɒmɪkəl/ *a.* 解剖的

accessory /ək'sesərɪ/ *a.* 附属的；辅助的

alimentary /ˌælɪ'mentərɪ/ *a.* 饮食的；消化的

esophagus /ɪ'sɒfəgəs/ *n.* 食管，食道

gallbladder /'gɔːlˌblædə/ *n.* 胆囊

moisten /'mɔɪsən/ *v.* 使湿润

diaphragm /'daɪəfræm/ *n.* 膈，横膈膜

diameter /daɪ'æmɪtə/ *n.* 直径

fundic /'fʌndɪk/ *a.* 基底的

duodenum /ˌdjuː'əˈdiːnəm/ *n.* 十二指肠

jejunum /dʒɪ'dʒuːnəm/ *n.* 空肠

bile /baɪl/ *n.* 胆汁

leftover /'leftəʊvə/ *n.* 剩余物

quadrant /'kwɒdrənt/ *n.* 四分体，象限

cecum /'siːkəm/ *n.* 盲肠

anal /'eɪnəl/ *a.* 肛门的

vermiform /'vɜːmɪfɔːm/ *a.* 蠕虫状的

bulk /bʌlk/ *n.* 体积；大块

transverse /'trænzvɜːs/ *a.* 横向的，横断的

sigmoid /'sɪgmɔɪd/ *a.* 乙状结肠的

exocrine /'eksəʊkrɪn/ *a.* 外分泌的

intercostal /ˌɪntə'kɒstəl/ *a.* 肋间的

glycogen /'glaɪkəʊdʒən/ *n.* 糖原

sac /sæk/ *n.* 囊

lobule /'lɒbjuːl/ *n.* 小叶

cholesterol /kə'lestərɒl/ *n.* 胆固醇

concentrated /'kɒnsənˌtreɪtɪd/ *a.* 浓缩的

disposal /dɪ'spəʊzəl/ *n.* 处理，处置

subdivision /ˌsʌbdɪ'vɪʒən/ *n.* 再分，细分

anus /'eɪnəs/ *n.* 肛门

pharynx /'færɪŋks/ *n.* 咽

salivary /'sælɪvərɪ/ *a.* 唾液的

uppermost /'ʌpəˌməʊst/ *a.* 最高的；最主要的

facilitate /fə'sɪlɪteɪt/ *v.* 促进；使容易

peristalsis /ˌperɪ'stælsɪs/ *n.* 蠕动

sphincter /'sfɪŋktə/ *n.* 括约肌

pyloric /paɪ'lɔːrɪk/ *a.* 幽门的

mesentery /'mesəntərɪ/ *n.* 肠系膜

ileum /'ɪlɪəm/ *n.* 回肠

mucus /'mjuːkəs/ *n.* 黏液

colon /'kəʊlən/ *n.* 结肠

peritoneal /ˌperɪtə'niːəl/ *a.* 腹膜的

rectum /'rektəm/ *n.* 直肠

pouch /paʊtʃ/ *n.* 囊，窝，陷凹

appendix /ə'pendɪks/ *n.* 阑尾；附录

ascend /ə'send/ *v.* 上升

descend /dɪ'send/ *v.* 下降，下行

flatten /'flætən/ *v.* 使变平

versatile /'vɜːsətɪl/ *a.* 万能的，通用的

carbohydrate /ˌkɑːbəʊ'haɪdreɪt/ *n.* 碳水化合物

detoxify /diː'tɒksɪfaɪ/ *v.* 使解毒

ventral /'ventrəl/ *a.* 腹部的

pigment /'pɪgmənt/ *n.* 色素

electrolyte /ɪ'lektrəlaɪt/ *n.* 电解质

▶ Notes

1.　该句是倒装句，其主语为 the pharynx，倒装是为了强调主语或避免主语部分过长导致句子头重脚轻。本句正常语序应为：The pharynx is just beyond the mouth, at the beginning of the tube leading to the stomach.。

2. simply put 意思是简言之，相当于 to put it in a simple way。

3. lining 此处指黏膜、壁，stomach lining 就是胃黏膜。相关短语 be lined with ... 常用来表示"以……作衬里"，"覆盖有……"。

4. detoxify 意为解毒，前缀 de- 在医学英语词汇中的应用非常广泛，可以用来表示向下、减少、降低、除去、否定、离开、解除、脱去等多种含义。例如：decompose（分解）、decompress（减压）、degeneration（退化）等。

5. lobule 指小叶，是由单词 lobe（叶）加上后缀 -ule 转变而来的。某些名词术语加上一定的后缀后，基本词义不变，专指形态较小的事物，这类后缀称为小词。例如：cellule（小细胞）、tubule（小管）、nodule（小结节）。类似的后缀还有 -let，如 platelet（血小板）。

Exercises

Ⅰ. **Choose the best answer to each of the following questions.**

1. Where is food stored for a short term after it is chewed?
    A. In the small intestine.   B. In the stomach.
    C. In the esophagus.   D. In the colon.

2. Why is the pharynx considered as a common passageway?
    A. Because it is for both respiration and voice production.
    B. Because it is for both digestion and food delivery.
    C. Because it is for both respiration and food digestion.
    D. Because it is for both voice production and digestion.

3. What determines the diameter of the stomach?
    A. The thickness of its wall.
    B. The amount of food it holds.
    C. The shape of its four regions.
    D. The size of the abdominal cavity.

4. The lower esophageal sphincter is surrounded by the _____.
    A. fundic region   B. pyloric region
    C. body region   D. cardiac region

5. The region that contributes to the entry of food to the duodenum is the _____.
    A. pyloric region   B. fundic region

C. body region   D. cardiac region

6. Which segments of the small intestine primarily perform the function of absorbing nutrients into the bloodstream?
   A. The jejunum and duodenum.
   B. The duodenum, jejunum and ileum.
   C. The duodenum and ileum.
   D. The jejunum and ileum.

7. What is the vermiform appendix attached to?
   A. The rectum.   B. The ascending colon.
   C. The cecum.   D. The duodenum.

8. What is the digestive gland that has both endocrine function and exocrine function?
   A. The pancreas.   B. The liver.
   C. The salivary glands.   D. The gallbladder.

9. Why is the liver described as the most versatile organ in the body?
   A. Because it is the largest gland in the body.
   B. Because it belongs to more than one system.
   C. Because it performs various functions.
   D. Because it works in conjunction with many other organs.

10. Where does the common bile duct open into?
    A. The hepatic lobules.   B. The duodenum.
    C. The jejunum.   D. The appendix.

Ⅱ. **Fill in each blank with a proper word mentioned in the text. The first letter of the word is given.**

1. A muscular tube that transports saliva, liquids, and foods is the e_____.

2. The muscle that separates the chest cavity from the abdomen is the d_____.

3. A series of muscle contractions that occur in the digestive tract are called p_____.

4. Bile is stored and concentrated in the g_____, a pear-shaped muscular sac.

5. The peritoneal fold attaching the small intestine to the posterior body wall is the m_____.

6. The worm-shaped pouch attached to the cecum is the a_____.

7. The distal portion of the small intestine is the i_____.

8. The principal sugar in blood serving as a major metabolic source of energy is g_____.

9. The large blind pouch forming the beginning of the large intestine is the c_____.

10. The l_____ is an important organ responsible for the normal metabolism of carbohydrates, fats, and proteins.

Ⅲ. **Fill in each blank in the following paragraph with a word in the box. Change the form of words if necessary.**

contraction	electrolyte	saliva	digestion	mucus
esophagus	mineral	colon	duodenum	breakdown
metabolism	relaxation	hormone	rectum	juice

Digestion involves the 1_____ of food into smaller and smaller components which can be absorbed and assimilated into the body. The secretion of 2_____ helps to produce a bolus（食团）which can be swallowed into the 3_____ to pass down into the stomach. Gastric 4_____ in the stomach is essential for the continuation of digestion as is the production of 5_____ in the stomach. Peristalsis is the rhythmic 6_____ of muscles that starts along the wall of the stomach. Most of the 7_____ of food takes place in the small intestine. Water and 8_____ are reabsorbed back into the blood, in the 9_____ of the large intestine. The waste products of digestion are removed from the anus via the 10_____.

Ⅳ. **Translate the following English sentences into Chinese.**

1. The digestive system is uniquely constructed to perform its specialized function of turning food into energy and packaging the residue for waste disposal.

2. Cells in the lining of the stomach secrete strong acid and powerful enzymes that are responsible for the breakdown process.

3. The small intestine is found in the central and lower portions of the abdominal cavity, where it is supported by a fan-shaped mesentery.

4. The most versatile organ in the body is the liver, which is also the largest gland in the body and situated high in the abdomen on the right side—often reaching the fourth intercostal space, under the diaphragm.

5. Bile, which contains salts, bile pigments, cholesterol, and electrolytes, becomes concentrated in the gallbladder as water is absorbed.

Ⅴ. **Write a 100-word summary of the properties and functions of the liver.**

Reading

Text B Diseases of the Digestive System and Their Treatment

Digestive diseases, also termed gastrointestinal diseases, are the diseases that affect the digestive system, which consists of the organs and pathways and processes responsible for processing food in the body.

Diseases of the Esophagus and Stomach

Gastroesophageal reflux disease (GERD) is a chronic symptom of **mucosal** damage caused by stomach acid coming up from the stomach into the esophagus. GERD usually develops from changes in the barrier between the stomach and the esophagus, including abnormal relaxation of the lower esophageal sphincter, which normally holds the top of the stomach closed, impaired **expulsion** of gastric reflux from the esophagus, or a **hiatal hernia**. These changes may be permanent or temporary. Treatment is typically via lifestyle changes and medications such as **proton** pump inhibitors, H2 receptor blockers, or **antacids**. Surgery may be an option in those who do not respond to medical **intervention**.

A **gastric ulcer** is an **erosion** or sore in the lining of the stomach that occurs when the protective mucus layer wears away[1] in certain areas, allowing damage to occur from the natural acids of the stomach. The majority of gastric ulcers are caused by bacteria called **Helicobacter pylori**[2] (H. pylori) or by taking **acetylsalicylic** acid or **non-steroidal** anti-inflammatory drugs (NSAID). Antibiotics are often used alone or in combination with **bismuth subsalicylate** in the treatment of gastric ulcers. **Neutralizing** or reducing stomach acid by taking drugs that directly inhibit the production of acid in the stomach promotes the healing of **peptic** ulcers regardless of the cause. In addition, it makes sense for people to keep away from foods that seem to **aggravate** pain and **bloating**. Eliminating possible stomach **irritants**, such as NSAIDs, alcohol, and **nicotine**, is also important.

Upper Gastrointestinal Hemorrhage

Upper gastrointestinal hemorrhage is commonly defined as bleeding arising from the esophagus, stomach, or duodenum. Blood may be observed in **hematemesis** or the altered form in the **stool** which is called **melena**. Depending on the severity of the blood loss, there may be symptoms of insufficient circulating blood volume and shock. Therefore, upper gastrointestinal bleeding is considered a medical emergency and typically requires hospital care for urgent diagnosis and treatment. Upper gastrointestinal bleeding can be induced by peptic ulcers, gastric erosions, esophageal **varices**[3], and some rarer causes such as gastric cancer. In line with[4] the source of bleeding, **endoscopic** therapy can be applied to reduce the risk of **recurrent** bleeding. If bleeding has ceased, the patient should be given oral iron and a normal diet. H2 blockade is usually **administered**[5] and may effectively reduce blood loss. Recurrent or refractory bleeding may lead to the need for surgery, although this has become uncommon as a result of improved endoscopic and medical treatment.

Diseases of the Small and Large Intestines

Appendicitis is a rather painful condition in which the fluid content of the appendix may increase to the point where it bursts. Many cases of appendicitis require removal of the **inflamed** appendix by **laparotomy** due to the high mortality associated with **rupture** of the appendix, which may give rise to severe **complications** such as **peritonitis** and **sepsis**.

Irritable bowel syndrome (IBS) is a collection of symptoms such as cramping, abdominal pain, bloating, diarrhea, and **constipation**. In spite of the **distress** it brings about, IBS does not **incur** serious diseases, such as cancer; neither does it permanently harm the large intestine. Most patients with IBS can ease symptoms with changes in diet, medicine, and stress relief.

Liver and Gallbladder Diseases

When a person is **afflicted** by a liver **ailment**, **jaundice** may occur. Jaundice is a **yellowish pigmentation** of the skin, the **conjunctival** membranes over the **sclera**, and other mucous membranes caused by increased levels of **bilirubin** in the blood. Jaundice, often a sign of **hepatitis** or liver cancer, may also indicate **leptospirosis** or obstruction of the **biliary** tract, such as **gallstones** or pancreatic cancer.

Hepatitis is a medical condition characterized by the presence of **inflammatory** cells in the tissue of the organ. In general, viral hepatitis occurs in several forms. Hepatitis A is usually acquired from drinking **sewage-contaminated** water.

Hepatitis B, which is usually spread by sexual contact, can also be transmitted by blood transfusions or contaminated needles. The hepatitis B virus is more contagious than the AIDS virus, which is spread in the same way. Thankfully, however, a vaccine is now available for hepatitis B. Hepatitis C, which is usually acquired by contact with infected blood and for which there is no vaccine, can lead to chronic hepatitis, liver cancer, and death.

As an irreversible result of various disorders that damage liver cells over time, **cirrhosis** is characterized by the replacement of liver tissue by fibrosis and **regenerative nodules**. Because of these changes, the liver function is eventually impaired. Despite the fact that cirrhosis is most commonly caused by hepatitis B, hepatitis C, **alcoholism**, and fatty liver disease, there are many other possible causes. Some cases of cirrhosis are idiopathic. **Ascites** is the most common complication of cirrhosis and it may be associated with a poor quality of life, increased risk of infection, or a poor long-term outcome. Other potentially life-threatening complications are hepatic **encephalopathy** and bleeding from esophageal varices. The treatment of cirrhosis usually focuses on preventing progression as well as complications. If liver damage progresses to liver failure, patients may be candidates for liver **transplantation**.

Cholecystitis occurs most commonly due to obstruction of the cystic duct with gallstones. Blockage of the cystic duct with gallstones causes accumulation of bile in the gallbladder and increased pressure within the gallbladder. Concentrated bile, pressure, and sometimes bacterial infection irritate and damage the gallbladder wall, causing inflammation and swelling of the gallbladder. Generally, females are twice as likely to develop cholecystitis as males. **Morbidity** and mortality may increase if the diagnosis of acute cholecystitis is delayed. **Uncomplicated** cholecystitis has an excellent **prognosis**; however, more than 25% of patients require surgery or develop complications.

▶ **Word Bank**

gastroesophageal /ˌgæstrəʊˌɪsɒfə'dʒiːəl/ *a.* 胃食管的

reflux /'riːflʌks/ *n.* 回流，反流

expulsion /ɪk'spʌlʃən/ *n.* 排出；呼出

hernia /'hɜːnɪə/ *n.* 疝

antacid /ænt'æsɪd/ *n.* 抗酸剂

gastric /'gæstrɪk/ *a.* 胃的

erosion /ɪ'rəʊʒən/ *n.* 侵蚀，腐蚀

pylorus /pə'lɔːrəs/ *n.* 幽门（复数为 pylori）

non-steroidal /ˌnɒnstɪə'rɔɪdəl/ *a.* 非甾体的

subsalicylate /ˌsʌbsə'lɪsəˌleɪt/ *n.* 碱式水杨酸盐

mucosal /mjuː'kəʊsəl/ *a.* 黏膜的

hiatal /haɪ'eɪtəl/ *a.* 裂孔的

proton /'prəʊtɒn/ *n.* 质子

intervention /ˌɪntə'venʃən/ *n.* 介入，干预

ulcer /'ʌlsə/ *n.* 溃疡

Helicobacter /ˌhelɪkəʊ'bæktə/ *n.* 螺杆菌

acetylsalicylic /ˌæsɪtɪlˌsæ'lɪsɪlɪk/ *a.* 乙酰水杨酸的

bismuth /'bɪzməθ/ *n.* 铋

neutralize /'njuːtrəlaɪz/ *v.* 中和

peptic /'peptɪk/ *a.* 消化的；胃蛋白酶的

bloating /'bləʊtɪŋ/ *n.* 鼓胀

nicotine /'nɪkəti:n/ *n.* 尼古丁

hematemesis /ˌhi:mə'teməsɪs/ *n.* 呕血

melena /mə'li:nə/ *n.* 黑便

endoscopic /ˌendə'skɒpɪk/ *a.* 内窥镜的

administer /əd'mɪnɪstə/ *v.* 给予（药物）

inflamed /ɪn'fleɪmd/ *a.* 发炎的；红肿的

rupture /'rʌptʃə/ *n.* 破裂

peritonitis /ˌperɪtə'naɪtɪs/ *n.* 腹膜炎

irritable /'ɪrɪtəbl/ *a.* 激惹性的

distress /dɪ'stres/ *n.* 痛苦

afflict /ə'flɪkt/ *v.* 困扰；折磨

jaundice /'dʒɔ:ndɪs/ *n.* 黄疸

pigmentation /ˌpɪgmen'teɪʃən/ *n.* 染色；色素沉积

sclera /'sklɪərə/ *n.* 巩膜

hepatitis /ˌhepə'taɪtɪs/ *n.* 肝炎

biliary /'bɪlɪərɪ/ *a.* 胆的；胆汁的

inflammatory /ɪn'flæmətərɪ/ *a.* 炎症的，发炎的

contaminate /kən'tæmɪneɪt/ *v.* 污染

regenerative /rɪ'dʒenərətɪv/ *a.* 再生的

alcoholism /'ælkəhɒˌlɪzəm/ *n.* 酗酒；酒精中毒

encephalopathy /enˌsefə'lɒpəθɪ/ *n.* 脑病

cholecystitis /ˌkəʊlɪsɪs'taɪtɪs/ *n.* 胆囊炎

uncomplicated /ʌn'kɒmplɪkeɪtɪd/ *a.* 无并发症的

aggravate /'ægrəveɪt/ *v.* 加重，使恶化

irritant /'ɪrɪtənt/ *n.* 刺激物

hemorrhage /'hemərɪdʒ/ *n.* 出血，失血

stool /stu:l/ *n.* 粪便

varix /'veərɪks/ *n.* 静脉曲张（复数为 varices）

recurrent /rɪ'kʌrənt/ *a.* 复发的

appendicitis /əˌpendə'saɪtɪs/ *n.* 阑尾炎

laparotomy /ˌlæpə'rɒtəmɪ/ *n.* 剖腹术

complication /ˌkɒmplɪ'keɪʃən/ *n.* 并发症

sepsis /'sepsɪs/ *n.* 败血症

constipation /ˌkɒnstɪ'peɪʃən/ *n.* 便秘

incur /ɪn'kɜ:/ *v.* 招致，引发

ailment /'eɪlmənt/ *n.* 小病

yellowish /'jeləʊɪʃ/ *a.* 微黄的，发黄的

conjunctival /ˌkɒndʒʌŋk'taɪvəl/ *a.* 结膜的

bilirubin /ˌbɪlɪ'ru:bɪn/ *n.* 胆红素

leptospirosis /ˌleptəʊspaɪə'rəʊsɪs/ *n.* 钩端螺旋体病

gallstone /'gɔ:lstəʊn/ *n.* 胆石

sewage /'su:ɪdʒ/ *n.* 污水

cirrhosis /sə'rəʊsɪs/ *n.* 肝硬化

nodule /'nɒdju:l/ *n.* 小结节，小瘤

ascites /æ'saɪtɪz/ *n.* 腹水

transplantation /ˌtrænzplɑ:n'teɪʃən/ *n.* 移植

morbidity /mɔ:'bɪdətɪ/ *n.* 发病率

prognosis /prɒg'nəʊsɪs/ *n.* 预后

▶ 注释

1. wear away 在该句中表示磨损。另外，wear away 还可以表示体力或勇气消耗殆尽，例如：The old woman has been worn away by her recent illness.（由于最近生病，老妇人的身体日趋衰弱。）。

2. pylori 是 pylorus 的复数形式，源于拉丁语。拉丁语中以 -us 结尾的名词变复数时将词尾变为 i。又如：bronchus（支气管）的复数是 bronchi，fungus（真菌）的复数是 fungi，bacillus（杆菌）的复数是 bacili，calculus（结石）的复数是calculi。

3. varices 是 varix 的复数形式，源于拉丁语。在拉丁语中，以 -ix 或者 -ex 结尾的名词变复数时结尾变成 -ices。又如：appendix（阑尾）的复数是 appendices，apex（尖端）的复数是 apices。

4. in line with 为介词短语，表示与……一致（相符），在该句中的意思是"根据……"。

5. administer 在该句中不是管理、执行的意思，而是表示给予（病人药物）。

Exercises

Ⅰ. **For each of the following statements, write "T" if the statement is true and "F" if the statement is false in the blank.**

_____ 1. Hiatal hernia is one of the common causes of gastroesophageal reflux disease.

_____ 2. Surgery is always the first option for those who have gastroesophageal reflux disease.

_____ 3. Bismuth subsalicylate is used alone in the treatment of gastric ulcers.

_____ 4. Hematemesis and melena are important signs suggesting upper gastrointestinal hemorrhage.

_____ 5. H2 blockade is clinically used to reduce upper gastrointestinal bleeding.

_____ 6. Jaundice may indicate hepatitis, liver cancer, leptospirosis, or obstruction of the biliary tract.

_____ 7. Hepatitis C is usually acquired from drinking sewage-contaminated water.

_____ 8. Endoscopic treatment becomes more common in the intervention of upper gastrointestinal hemorrhage.

_____ 9. Cirrhosis is characterized by the replacement of liver tissue by fibrosis and regenerative nodules.

_____ 10. If liver damage progresses to ascites, patients may need liver transplantation.

Ⅱ. **Match each term in Column A with its corresponding description in Column B. Write the corresponding letter in the blank.**

Column A	Column B
_____ 1. reflux	A. prediction of the probable course and outcome of a disease
_____ 2. ulcer	B. infrequent or incomplete bowel movements
_____ 3. hematemesis	C. the formation of fibrous tissue
_____ 4. melena	D. inflammatory lesion through skin or mucous membrane resulting from necrosis (坏死) of tissue
_____ 5. laparotomy	E. the passage of dark stools containing blood
_____ 6. constipation	F. the backward flow of fluid in the body
_____ 7. fibrosis	G. a severe liver disease characterized by the replacement of liver tissues by fibrosis and regenerative nodules
_____ 8. cirrhosis	H. inflammation of the gallbladder wall
_____ 9. cholecystitis	I. a surgical procedure that involves incision into the abdominal cavity
_____ 10. prognosis	J. the vomiting of blood

Ⅲ. **Translate the following Chinese sentences into English.**

1. 无论是何种原因引起的胃溃疡，通过服用抑酸药以中和或减少胃酸分泌，有助于促进消化性溃疡的愈合。

2. 由于阑尾穿孔引起的高死亡率，很多阑尾炎患者需行阑尾切除术，开腹切除炎症阑尾。

3. 尽管肠易激综合征给患者带来痛苦，但它并不会诱发癌症等严重疾病，也不会长期损害大肠。

4. 腹水是肝硬化最常见的并发症，可能导致患者生存质量下降、感染风险增加或长期预后不良。

5. 胆汁浓缩、压力增高、细菌感染均可刺激并损伤胆囊壁，引起胆囊炎症和胆囊肿胀。

Ⅳ. **Think critically and then answer the following questions.**

1. A 7-year-old girl presented to the emergency department with a chief

complaint of mid-abdominal pain for one day. The pain started after lunch yesterday. This was followed by vomiting, which did not relieve the pain. She did not feel like eating dinner. By this morning the pain increased and she vomited again. The pain has moved to the right lower abdomen. What might be the little girl's problem? What is the most effective management of this disorder?

2. A 35-year-old man who went to see a physician stated that he had had a gastric ulcer three years before and that recently he noticed an increased dull pain in his stomach and back. Besides, he had heartburn and belched (打嗝) a lot. What might be responsible for his disorder? What should be the goal of treatment?

Medicine in China

Liver Surgery Pioneer

Wu Mengchao (1922–2021) is known as China's "father of Chinese hepatobiliary surgery".

Wu was born in 1922 into a poor family in Minqing county, Fujian Province. In 1949, he graduated from the Tongji University School of Medicine in Shanghai. Despite his diminutive height of 1.6 meters, Wu was a towering figure in China's medical community and was widely celebrated for his pioneering spirit and bold ingenuity, even in difficult economic and social circumstances.

China in the 1950s had no theoretical basis or clinical research in liver surgery. In 1956, Wu heard from a colleague that a visiting Japanese surgeon said it would take at least 30 years for China to catch up with the rest of the world. "I wasn't pleased hearing this comment, so I made it my mission to propel China's liver and gallbladder surgery into the front-runners of the world," he said.

Two years later, Wu published the country's first basic textbook on liver surgery which he had translated from English into Chinese. During that period, he was sometimes ill with severe dysentery, but this did not hinder his translation work.

In 1960, Wu came up with a revolutionary approach that divided a liver's anatomy into "five lobes and four segments", a significant improvement from the dual lobes model used by Chinese physicians in the past. The same year, Wu successfully performed the first liver surgery in China. In the 1980s, he perfected a new technique of vascular inflow occlusion that can be performed at room temperature, instead of in controlled conditions. The technique involves clamping the hepatic vein and artery to reduce blood loss and protect liver tissue during surgery, a technique still used by surgeons around the globe today.

In 1991, Wu was elected an academician of the Chinese Academy of Sciences. In 2005, he became the first physician to receive the State Preeminent Science and Technology Award, China's highest academic award, for raising the completion rate of successful hepatic surgery for liver cancer patients in China from 16 percent to over 98 percent.

During seven decades' practice in medicine, Wu conducted more than 16,000 operations and saved nearly 20,000 lives. He retired in 2019 at the age of 97, becoming the world's longest active liver surgeon.

Exercises

Ⅰ. **Translate the underlined part into Chinese.**

Ⅱ. **Answer the following question.**

What good qualities did Wu Mengchao have as a surgeon?

Chapter 7

Cardiovascular System

Pre-Reading Question

What is the meaning of "One's heart misses a beat"? On what occasion would your heart miss a beat?

Reading

Text A Structure and Functions of the Cardiovascular System

The cardiovascular system consists of the heart, blood vessels, and approximately 5 liters of blood that the blood vessels transport. Responsible for[1] transporting oxygen, nutrients, hormones, and cellular waste products throughout the body, the cardiovascular system is powered by the body's hardest-working organ—the heart.

The heart weighs between 200 and 425 grams and is a little larger than the size of your fist. By the end of a long life, a person's heart may have beaten (expanded and contracted) more than 3.5 billion times. In fact, each day the average heart beats 100,000 times, pumping about 2,000 **gallons** (7,571 liters) of blood.

The heart lies within the **mediastinum** (in the thoracic cavity **cradled** between the lungs, just behind the sternum). The bottom tip of the heart, known as its **apex**, is turned to the left so that about two-thirds of the heart is located on the left side of the body with the other one-third on the right.[2] The top of the heart, known as the **base** of the heart, connects to the great blood vessels of the body: the **aorta**, **vena cava**, **pulmonary** artery, and pulmonary **veins** (Figure 7-1).

A double-layered membrane called **pericardium** surrounds your heart like a sac. The outer layer of the pericardium surrounds the roots of the major blood vessels of your heart and is attached by ligaments to your spinal column, diaphragm, and other parts of your body. The inner layer of the pericardium is attached to the heart muscle. A coating of fluid separates the two layers of membrane, letting the heart move as it beats, yet still be attached to your body.[3]

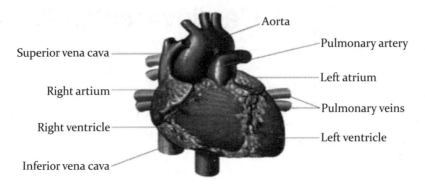

Figure 7-1   Heart anatomy

The heart has four **chambers**. The upper chambers are called the left and right atria, and the lower chambers are called the left and right ventricles. A wall of muscle called the **septum** separates the left and right atria and the left and right ventricles. The left ventricle is the largest and strongest chamber in your heart. The walls of the left ventricle are only about half an inch thick, but they have enough force to push blood through the **aortic** valve and into your body.

Four types of valves regulate blood flow through your heart: The **tricuspid** valve regulates blood flow between the right atrium and the right ventricle. The pulmonary **semilunar** valve controls blood flow from the right ventricle into the pulmonary arteries, which carry blood to your lungs to pick up oxygen. The **mitral** valve lets oxygen-rich blood from your lungs pass from the left atrium into the left ventricle. The aortic valve opens the way for oxygen-rich blood to pass from the left ventricle into the aorta, the largest artery of your body, where it is delivered to the rest of your body.

There are two primary **circulatory loops** in the human body: the pulmonary circulation loop and the systemic circulation loop. Pulmonary circulation transports **deoxygenated** blood from the right atrium and the right ventricle to the lungs, and returns **oxygenated** (oxygen-rich) blood back to the left atrium of the heart. Systemic circulation carries highly oxygenated blood from the left atrium and the left ventricle to the aorta which branches into arteries to distribute freshly oxygenated blood to each part of the body, to remove wastes from body tissues, and to return deoxygenated blood to the right side of the heart.

Electrical impulses from your heart muscle (myocardium) cause your heart to beat (contract). These electrical signals begin in the **sinoatrial** (SA) **node**, located at the top of the right atrium. The SA node is sometimes called the "natural pacemaker" of the heart. When an electrical impulse is released from this natural pacemaker, it causes the atria to contract. The signal then passes through the **atrioventricular** (AV) node. The AV node **checks** the signal and sends it through muscle fibers of the ventricles, causing them to contract. The SA node sends electrical impulses at a certain rate, but your heart rate may still change, depending on physical demands, stress, or **hormonal** factors.[4]

A heartbeat is a two-phase pumping action that takes about a second. These phases are called **diastole** (relaxation) and **systole** (contraction). Diastole occurs when ventricle walls relax and the blood flows into the heart from the venae cavae and the pulmonary veins. The tricuspid and mitral valves are open in diastole, as blood passes from the right and left atria into the ventricles. The pulmonary and aortic valves are closed during diastole. Systole occurs next, as the walls of the right and left ventricles contract to pump blood into the pulmonary artery and the aorta. Both the tricuspid and mitral valves are closed during systole, thus preventing the flow of blood back into the atria.[5]

All blood vessels are lined with[6] a thin layer of simple **squamous** epithelium known as the **endothelium** that keeps blood cells inside the blood vessels and prevents **clots** from forming. There are three major types of blood vessels: arteries, **capillaries**, and veins. Arteries are blood vessels that carry oxygenated blood away from the heart to the tissues of the body. Arteries face high levels of blood pressure as they carry blood being pushed from the heart under great force. To **withstand** this pressure, the walls of the arteries are thicker, more **elastic**, and more muscular than those of other vessels. **Arterioles** are narrower arteries that branch off from the ends of arteries and carry blood to capillaries. Capillaries are the smallest and thinnest of blood vessels in the body and also the most common. They connect to arterioles on one end and **venules** on the other. Capillaries carry blood very close to the cells or the tissues of the body in order to exchange gases, nutrients, and waste products. Veins are thinner-walled than arteries. They conduct blood toward the heart from the tissues. Veins have little elastic tissue and less connective tissue than arteries, and blood pressure in veins is extremely low. Veins have valves that prevent the backflow of blood and keep blood moving in one direction.

The cardiovascular system has three major functions: transportation of materials, protection from pathogens, and regulation of the homeostasis of the body. 1) *Transportation*: The cardiovascular system transports essential nutrients and oxygen to and removes wastes and carbon dioxide from the tissues of the body. 2) *Protection*: The cardiovascular system protects the body through its white blood cells. White blood cells clean up cellular **debris** and fight pathogens that have entered the body. **Platelets** and red blood cells form **scabs** to seal wounds and prevent pathogens from entering the body and liquids from leaking out.

3) *Regulation*: The cardiovascular system is **instrumental** in the body's ability to maintain **homeostatic** control of several internal conditions. Blood vessels near the surface of the skin open during **overheating** to allow hot blood to **dump** its heat into the body's surroundings. Blood also helps balance the pH in the body due to the presence of **bicarbonate** ions, which act as a **buffer** solution.

It is important to maintain a healthy cardiovascular system since the blood and blood vessels are crucial to good health. The cardiovascular system is the **workhorse** of the body, continuously moving to push blood to the cells. If this important system ceases its work, the body dies.

▶ Word Bank

gallon /'gælən/ *n.* 加仑（容量单位）

cradle /'kreɪdl/ *v.* 怀抱

base /beɪs/ *n.* 心底

vena cava /'viːnə 'keɪvə/ *n.* 腔静脉（复数为 venae canae）

pulmonary /'pʌlmənərɪ/ *a.* 肺的；肺动脉的

pericardium /ˌperɪ'kɑːdɪəm/ *n.* 心包膜，心包

septum /'septəm/ *n.* 隔膜

tricuspid /traɪ'kʌspɪd/ *a.* 三尖的

mitral /'maɪtrəl/ *a.* 二尖的

loop /luːp/ *n.* 回路

oxygenate /'ɒksɪdʒɪneɪt/ *v.* 含氧

node /nəʊd/ *n.* 节点，结节

check /tʃek/ *v.* 阻止

diastole /daɪ'æstəlɪ/ *n.* 心脏舒张期

squamous /'skweɪməs/ *a.* 有鳞的，多鳞的；鳞状的

clot /klɒt/ *n.* 凝块，阻塞

withstand /wɪð'stænd/ *v.* 经得起，承受

arteriole /ɑː'tɪərɪəʊl/ *n.* 小动脉，细动脉

debris /'debriː/ *n.* 碎片，残骸

scab /skæb/ *n.* 痂，疥癣

homeostatic /ˌhəʊmɪə'stætɪk/ *a.* 体内平衡的

dump /dʌmp/ *v.* 抛弃；排出

buffer /'bʌfə/ *n.* 缓冲；*v.* 缓冲；减轻

mediastinum /ˌmiːdɪæ'staɪnəm/ *n.* 纵隔

apex /'eɪpeks/ *n.* 心尖；顶点

aorta /eɪ'ɔːtə/ *n.* 主动脉

vein /veɪn/ *n.* 静脉

chamber /'tʃeɪmbə/ *n.* 室，房间

aortic /eɪ'ɔːtɪk/ *a.* 主动脉的

semilunar /ˌsemɪ'luːnə/ *a.* 半月形的

circulatory /ˌsɜːkjʊ'leɪtərɪ/ *a.* 循环的

deoxygenate /diː'ɒksɪdʒɪneɪt/ *v.* 脱氧

sinoatrial /ˌsaɪnəʊ'eɪtrɪəl/ *a.* 窦房的

atrioventricular /ˌeɪtrɪəʊven'trɪkjʊlə/ *a.* 房室的

hormonal /hɔː'məʊnəl/ *a.* 荷尔蒙的，激素的

systole /'sɪstəlɪ/ *n.* 心脏收缩期

endothelium /ˌendəʊ'θiːlɪəm/ *n.* 内皮细胞层

capillary /'kæpɪlərɪ/ *n.* 毛细血管；*a.* 毛细管的

elastic /ɪ'læstɪk/ *a.* 灵活的，有弹性的

venule /'venjuːl/ *n.* 小静脉

platelet /'pleɪtlɪt/ *n.* 血小板

instrumental /ˌɪnstrə'mentəl/ *a.* 有帮助的

overheating /ˌəʊvə'hiːtɪŋ/ *n.* 过热

bicarbonate /baɪ'kɑːbənət/ *n.* 碳酸氢根

workhorse /'wɜːkhɔːs/ *n.* 重负荷机器

▶ Notes

1. responsible for 这个形容词短语在句中充当原因状语。形容词短语可在句中当伴随、时间、原因状语。需要注意的是，形容词短语的逻辑主语应和句子主语

一致，否则不能用此结构，如：Eager to improve his body condition, he faithfully complied with the doctor's advice.（他急切地想改善自己的身体状况，所以严格遵照医生的医嘱），又如：Unable to contract efficiently, the ventricles fail to pump a sufficient amount of blood required by the human body.（心室不能有效收缩，就不能泵出人体所需的充足的血量）。

2. with the other one-third on the right 是一个省略结构，完整形式为：with the other one-third of the heart located on the right side of the body。由于 with 前后结构相同，用词也一样，所以省略了重复的词语。

3. 该句子中现在分词短语 letting the heart move as it beats 是句子的伴随状语，它的逻辑主语是 a coating of fluid。yet still be attached to the body 结构与省略了 to 的不定式短语 move as it beats 并列，共同作 let the heart 的宾语补足语。

4. 该句中分词短语 depending on 作句子的状语，表示依……而定；因……而异。医学文献中常用 depending on 这个短语来表达不同情况应采用不同措施策略的含义。如：Treatment includes antibiotics or simply supportive care, depending on cause and severity.（治疗依病因和症状严重程度而定，可采取抗菌素和支持疗法。）。

5. 该句中副词 thus + 现在分词作结果状语，意思是从而、借此，如：The universities have expanded, thus giving many more people the opportunity to receive higher education.（大学扩招了，这样就使更多人有机会接受高等教育）。

6. be lined with 表示用……衬里、覆盖。在医学文献中，该词组常用于表示内膜上衬有、布满，如：The walls of the sinuses are lined with endocytic cells which engulf any foreign particles that might be present in the lymph.（窦壁上布满了内吞细胞，这些细胞能吞噬淋巴中可能出现的任何一种外来颗粒）。

Exercises

Ⅰ. **Choose the best answer to each of the following questions.**

1. What is the bottom tip of the heart called?
   A. The sternum.　　　　　　　B. The base.
   C. The apex.　　　　　　　　D. The aorta.

2. The fluid-filled sac that surrounds the heart and keeps it contained within the chest cavity is the _____.
   A. pericardium　　　　　　　B. myocardium
   C. endocardium　　　　　　　D. diaphragm

3. What happens in the pulmonary circulation loop?
   A. Deoxygenated blood is carried from the lungs to the heart.

B. Deoxygenated blood is carried from the heart to the lungs.

C. Oxygenated blood is carried from the lungs to the heart.

D. Oxygenated blood is carried from the heart to the lungs.

4. In the cardiac cycle, the tricuspid valve prevents blood from flowing back into the _____.

A. right atrium   B. left atrium

C. aorta   D. left ventricle

5. What function does the atrioventricular node perform?

A. Causing the atria to contract.

B. Initiating the electrical impulse.

C. Regulating the natural heartbeat.

D. Causing the ventricles to contract.

6. During _____ of the cardiac cycle, the atria and ventricles are relaxed, and deoxygenated blood from the venae cavae flows into the right atrium.

A. systole phase   B. pumping phase

C. diastole phase   D. respiration phase

7. When ventricles contract to pump blood into the pulmonary artery and the aorta, _____.

A. the pulmonary and mitral valves are open

B. the pulmonary and aortic valves are closed

C. the tricuspid and mitral valves are closed

D. the tricuspid and aortic valves are open

8. Why are the walls of arteries thicker than those of other blood vessels?

A. Because the thick walls can prevent blood from leaking out of vessels.

B. Because the thick walls can keep clots from forming.

C. Because the thick walls can conduct a larger volume of blood.

D. Because the thick walls can bear high pressure of the blood from the heart.

9. Which type of blood vessels directly exchange gases, nutrients, and waste products with body tissues?

A. The arterioles.   B. The capillaries.

C. The veins.   D. The venules.

10. Platelets can help the human body to _____.

A. form scabs to stop bleeding

B. remove cellular wastes from the body

C. attack the pathogens that enter into the body

D. keep the balance of several internal conditions

Ⅱ . **Write the names of the arrow-indicated parts of the heart in the spaces given.**

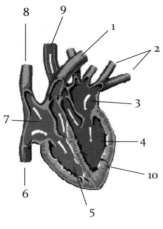

1. _____   2. _____

3. _____   4. _____

5. _____   6. _____

7. _____   8. _____

9. _____   10. _____

Ⅲ . **Fill in each blank in the following paragraph with a word in the box. Change the form of words if necessary.**

vein	heartbeat	capillary	septum	stomach
artery	abdominal	wall	pump	chamber
lung	deoxygenate	pulse	thoracic	heart

Your heart and circulatory system make up your cardiovascular system. The heart is a four- 1_____ "double pump," where each side (left and right) operates as a separate pump. It is located medial (中间的) to the 2_____ along the body's midline in the 3_____ region. The left and right sides of the heart are separated by a 4_____ of separated tissue known as the 5_____ of the heart. The right side of the heart receives 6_____ blood from the systemic 7_____ and pumps it to the lungs for oxygenation. The left side of the heart receives oxygenated blood from the lungs and pumps it through the systemic 8_____ to the tissues of the body. Each results in the simultaneous（同时的）9_____ of both sides of the heart, making the 10_____ a very efficient pump.

Ⅳ. Translate the following English sentences into Chinese.

1. A coating of fluid separates the two layers of membrane, letting the heart move as it beats, yet still be attached to your body.

2. The aortic valve opens the way for oxygen-rich blood to pass from the left ventricle into the aorta, the largest artery of your body, where it is delivered to the rest of your body.

3. The AV node checks the signal and sends it through muscle fibers of the ventricles, causing them to contract.

4. All blood vessels are lined with a thin layer of simple squamous epithelium known as the endothelium that keeps blood cells inside the blood vessels and prevents clots from forming.

5. The cardiovascular system transports essential nutrients and oxygen to and removes wastes and carbon dioxide from the tissues of the body.

Ⅴ. Write a 100-word summary to explain how the heart valves work to complete the pulmonary circulation.

Reading

Text B   Diseases of the Cardiovascular System and Their Treatment

The pathological conditions of the cardiovascular system are grouped into four categories: pathological conditions of the heart, pathological conditions of the blood vessels, congenital heart diseases, and **arrhythmia**.

Pathological Conditions of the Heart

Coronary artery disease is usually the result of atherosclerosis. This is the **deposition** of fatty **compounds** on the inner lining of the coronary arteries. The ordinarily smooth lining of the artery becomes **roughened** as the **atherosclerotic** plaque collects in the artery. Atherosclerosis is dangerous for two important reasons. First, narrowing of the vessel due to atherosclerosis can cause inflexibility and plugging up of the vessel. Second, the roughened lining of the artery may rupture or cause abnormal clotting of blood, leading to a **thrombotic occlusion**.

In both cases, blood flow decreases or stops entirely, leading to **necrosis** of a part of the myocardium. The area of dead myocardial tissue is known as **infarction**. The infarcted area is eventually replaced by scar tissue. Accepted treatments for **occluded** coronary arteries include medications, **percutaneous transluminal** coronary **angioplasty**, directional coronary **atherectomy**, and coronary **bypass** surgery.

Angina pectoris, also called angina, is caused by an insufficient supply of blood to the myocardium. Angina attacks are frequently triggered by conditions that increase the oxygen demand of the myocardium, such as **exertion** or stress. Angina is not technically a disease, but rather a symptom of coronary artery disease.[1] For acute attacks of angina, **nitroglycerin** is given **sublingually**[2]. This drug, one of several drugs called **nitrates**, is a powerful **vasodilator** and muscle **relaxant**.

Congestive heart failure occurs when the heart is unable to pump its required amount of blood (more blood enters the heart from the veins than leaves through the arteries).[3] Blood accumulates in the lungs, causing pulmonary **edema**. Damming back of blood resulting from right-sided heart failure results in the accumulation of fluid in the abdominal organs and **subcutaneous** tissue of the legs.[4] Congestive heart failure often develops gradually over several years, although it can be acute. Therapy includes lowering dietary intake of **sodium** and taking **diuretics** to promote loss of fluids.

Endocarditis refers to the inflammation of the membrane lining of the valves and chambers of the heart caused by direct invasion of bacteria or other organisms, leading to deformity of the valve **cusps**. Damage to the heart valves may cause lesions called **vegetations** that may break off into the bloodstream, forming **emboli** that **lodge** in other organs. If the emboli lodge in the small vessels of the skin, multiple **pinpoint** hemorrhages called **petechiae** may appear. Antibiotics are effective in curing bacterial endocarditis. Therapy will likely continue over the course of several weeks.

Pericarditis is usually caused by bacterial infection of the pericardium surrounding the heart. In most cases, pericarditis is **secondary** to disease elsewhere in the body (such as pulmonary infection). **Malaise**, fever, and chest pain occur, and fluid accumulates within the **pericardial** cavity. Compression of the heart due to collection of fluid is called cardiac **tamponade**. If a considerable amount of fluid is present, pressure on the pulmonary veins may slow the return of blood from the lungs. Excess liquid is drained by **pericardiocentesis**.

Rheumatic heart disease is caused by rheumatic fever. Rheumatic fever is a disease that usually occurs in childhood and can follow a few weeks after a **streptococcal** infection. Damage is done to the heart, particularly the heart valves, by one or more attacks of rheumatic fever. The valves, especially the mitral valve, become **inflamed** and scarred, so they do not open and close normally. Treatment consists of reduced activity, drugs to control arrhythmia, surgery to repair or replace a damaged valve, and **anticoagulant** therapy to prevent emboli from forming.

Pathological Conditions of the Blood Vessels

Aneurysm is a localized **dilatation** of an artery formed at a weak point in the vessel wall. This weakened area **balloons** out with each **pulsation** of the artery. The danger of an aneurysm is that as the wall of the artery pushes outward, it becomes progressively thinner and may eventually rupture, leading to hemorrhage and ultimately death. Treatment of an aneurysm depends on the particular vessel involved. In aneurysms of small vessels in the brain (berry aneurysms), treatment is occlusion of the vessel with small **clips**. For larger arteries, such as the aorta, the aneurysm is **resected** and a **synthetic graft** is sewn within the aneurysm.

Hypertension is a condition in which the patient has a higher blood pressure than that judged to be normal.[5] Most high blood pressure is **essential** hypertension, in which the cause of the increased pressure is idiopathic. In adults, a blood pressure equal to or greater than 140/90 mmHg is considered high. Diuretics, **beta-blockers**, **ACE** inhibitors, and calcium channel blockers are used as treatment for essential hypertension. Losing weight, limiting sodium intake, and reducing fat in the diet are also important in therapy. In secondary hypertension, there are always some associated lesions, such as **glomerulonephritis**, or disease of the adrenal glands, which is responsible for the elevated blood pressure.

Congenital Heart Diseases

Tetralogy of Fallot, named after[6] French physician Étienne-Louis-Arthur-Fallot[7], is a congenital heart **anomaly** that consists of four defects: pulmonary **stenosis**, **interventricular septal** defect, shift of the aorta to the right, and **hypertrophy** of the right ventricles. An infant with this condition is described as a "blue baby" because of the extreme degree of **cyanosis** present at birth. Surgery is required to repair the various heart defects.

Coarctation of the aorta is a congenital heart defect characterized by a localized narrowing of the aorta, which results in increased blood pressure in the upper extremities and decreased blood pressure in the lower extremities. Surgical correction of the defect is **curative** if the disease is diagnosed early.

Patent ductus arteriosus is an abnormal opening between the pulmonary artery and the aorta caused by failure of the fetal ductus arteriosus to close after birth. This defect is seen primarily in premature infants. Treatment is surgically closing the ductus arteriosus.

Arrhythmia

Heart **block** is the failure of proper conduction of impulses through the AV node to the atrioventricular **bundle**. Damage to the SA node may cause its impulses to be too weak to activate the AV node and the impulses fail to reach the ventricles. If the failure occurs only occasionally, the heart will miss a beat in a rhythm at regular intervals. **Implantation** of a cardiac pacemaker can overcome heart block and establish a normal rhythm.

Atrial **fibrillation** is extremely rapid, incomplete contractions of the atria resulting in disorganized and uncoordinated **twitching** of the atria. At these rapid rates, the ventricles cannot contract efficiently or recover adequately between contractions. These inefficient contractions of the heart reduce the blood flow, leading to angina and congestive heart failure. In order to restore normal heart rhythm, an electrical device called a **defibrillator** is applied to the chest wall to **reverse** its abnormal rhythm.

▶ Word Bank

arrhythmia /əˈrɪθmɪə/ n. 心律不齐，节律失调

compound /ˈkɒmpaʊnd/ n. 化合物，复合物

atherosclerotic /ˌæθərəʊskləˈrɒtɪk/ a. 动脉粥样硬化的

occlusion /əˈkluːʒən/ n. 闭塞，梗塞

infarction /ɪnˈfɑːkʃən/ n. 梗死

percutaneous /ˌpɜːkjuːˈteɪnɪəs/ a. 经由皮肤的

transluminal /trænsˈluːmɪnəl/ a. 经腔的；穿过（血管）壁的

angioplasty /ˈændʒɪəʊˌplæstɪ/ n. 血管成形术，血管修复术

atherectomy /ˌæðɪˈrektəmɪ/ n. 经皮腔内斑块旋切术

angina pectoris /ænˈdʒaɪnə ˈpektərɪs/ n. 心绞痛

nitroglycerin /ˌnaɪtrəʊˈglɪsərɪn/ n. 硝酸甘油

nitrate /ˈnaɪtreɪt/ n. 硝酸盐

relaxant /rɪˈlæksənt/ n. 松弛剂

edema /ɪˈdiːmə/ n. 浮肿，水肿

sodium /ˈsəʊdɪəm/ n. 钠

endocarditis /ˌendəʊkɑːˈdaɪtɪs/ n. 心内膜炎

vegetation /ˌvedʒəˈteɪʃən/ n. 赘生物，赘疣

embolus /ˈembələs/ n. 栓子，栓塞物（复数为 emboli）

lodge /lɒdʒ/ v. 存放；滞留

petechia /pɪˈtiːkɪə/ n. 瘀点，瘀斑（复数为 petechiae）

pericarditis /ˌperɪkɑːˈdaɪtɪs/ n. 心包炎

deposition /ˌdepəˈzɪʃən/ n. 沉积

roughen /ˈrʌfən/ v. 使粗糙

thrombotic /θrɒmˈbɒtɪk/ a. 血栓形成的

necrosis /neˈkrəʊsɪs/ n. 坏死

occlude /əˈkluːd/ v. 使闭塞，封闭

bypass /ˈbaɪpɑːs/ n. 支路，旁道

exertion /ɪgˈzɜːʃən/ n. 用力，费力

sublingually /ˈsʌblɪŋgwəlɪ/ ad. 舌下（地）

vasodilator /ˌvæsəʊdaɪˈleɪtə/ n. 血管舒张药

congestive /kənˈdʒestɪv/ a. 充血的

subcutaneous /ˌsʌbkjʊˈteɪnɪəs/ a. 皮下的

diuretic /daɪˈjʊəretɪk/ n. 利尿剂，利尿药

cusp /ˈkʌsp/ n. 尖头，尖端

pinpoint /ˈpɪnpɔɪnt/ n. 针尖；微小之物

secondary /ˈsekəndərɪ/ a. 继发的

malaise /mə'leɪz/ *n.* 身体不适

pericardial /ˌperɪ'kɑːdɪəl/ *a.* 心包的

tamponade /ˌtæmpə'neɪd/ *n.* 填塞，压塞

pericardiocentesis /'perɪˌkɑːdɪəʊsen'tiːsɪs/ *n.* 心包（放液）穿刺术

rheumatic /rʊ'mætɪk/ *a.* 风湿症的；风湿症引起的

streptococcal /ˌstreptə'kɒkəl/ *a.* 链状球菌的；链球菌导致的

inflame /ɪn'fleɪm/ *v.* 发炎；加剧

anticoagulant /ˌæntɪkəʊ'ægjʊlənt/ *a.* 抗凝的

aneurysm /'ænjʊrɪzəm/ *n.* 动脉瘤

dilatation /ˌdɪlə'teɪʃən/ *n.* 膨胀，扩张

balloon /bə'luːn/ *v.* 使膨胀

pulsation /pʌl'seɪʃən/ *n.* 脉动，博动

clip /klɪp/ *n.* 夹子，钳

resect /rɪ'sekt/ *v.* 切除，割除

synthetic /sɪn'θetɪk/ *a.* 合成的，人造的

graft /grɑːft/ *n.* 移植，移植物

essential /ɪ'senʃəl/ *a.* 原发的

beta-blocker /'beɪtə 'blɒkə/ *n.* β– 阻断剂，β– 受体阻断药

ACE (angiotensin-converting enzyme 的缩写) 血管紧张素转换酶

glomerulonephritis /gləʊˌmerjʊləʊne'fraɪtɪs/ *n.* 肾小球性肾炎

tetralogy /te'trælədʒɪ/ *n.* 四联症

anomaly /ə'nɒməlɪ/ *n.* 异常，反常

stenosis /stɪ'nəʊsɪs/ *n.* 狭窄

interventricular /ˌɪntəven'trɪkjʊlə/ *a.* （心脏）室间的

septal /'septəl/ *a.* 隔膜的，中隔的

hypertrophy /haɪ'pɜːtrəfɪ/ *n.* 肥大，过度生长

cyanosis /ˌsaɪə'nəʊsɪs/ *n.* 紫绀

coarctation /ˌkəʊɑːk'teɪʃən/ *n.* 狭窄，收缩

curative /'kjʊərətɪv/ *a.* 有治病效力的

patent /'pætənt/ *a.* 开放的，不闭合的

ductus /'dʌktəs/ *n.* 导管

arteriosus /ɑːˌtɪəriː'əʊsəs/ *a.* 动脉的

block /blɒk/ *n.* 阻滞

bundle /'bʌndl/ *n.* 束，捆

implantation /ˌɪmplɑːn'teɪʃən/ *n.* 植入，移植；着床

fibrillation /ˌfɪbrɪ'leɪʃən/ *n.* 纤维性颤动；纤颤

twitching /'twɪtʃɪŋ/ *n.* 抽动，痉挛

defibrillator /diː'fɪbrɪleɪtə/ *n.* 除颤器

reverse /rɪ'vɜːs/ *v.* 逆转，倒退

▶ Notes

1. 该句中 not ... , but rather ... 表示"不是……，而是……"。 not ... , but ... 结构也表示"不是……，而是……"的意思，在 but 后添加副词 rather 起加强语气作用，更强烈地表示与前分句的对比意味，如：The patient was no better but rather grew worse.（病人的情况不但没有见好，反而恶化了）。

2. be given sublingually 表示舌下给药。给药方式多用副词或介词短语表示。例如：be given orally"口服"，intravenously"静脉内给药"，intramuscularly"肌内给药"，subcutaneously "皮下给药"，submucously "黏膜下给药"，by intramuscular injection "肌肉注射"，by intravenous infusion (perfusion) "静脉输注"，by aerosol "喷雾给药"，by enema "灌肠"，per rectum "直肠给药"。

3. 该句中 than 后省略主语 blood。当这种结构中 than 前后句子的主语相同时，可省略主语。若 than 前后谓语相同，可以省略谓语动词或用 do 代替，如：

The blood substitutes have a greater ability to release oxygen to the tissues than red blood cells (do).（血液替代品为组织释放氧气的能力要强于血红细胞）。若比较结构 than 前后句子表语相同，可以省略表语，如：Red blood cells are much more common than the other blood particles.（血红细胞要比其他血液粒子更常见。），这里 blood particles 后省略了 are common。

4. 该句中现在分词短语 resulting from 作主语 damming back of blood 的定语。另外，还应注意词组 result in 和 result from 的区别：result in 表示导致……结果，后加结果。result from 表示由……导致，后加原因。

5. 该句的比较结构中省略了一些成分，补全后完整的句子是 The patient has a higher blood pressure than the blood pressure judged to be normal.。课文中用 that 替换 the blood pressure，以避免重复，使句子更加简练。需要注意的是，用 that 或 those 替换名词时，它们总是伴随着限定性的后置修饰语，如：The number of vessels examined in the present study was considerably less than *that* measured in the previous studies.（本研究测定的血管数要远远少于之前研究中测量的血管数）。

6. name after 这个短语动词表示以……命名，又如：Parkinson's disease was named after the English doctor James Parkinson, who was the first to report on the disease.（帕金森病是以最先报告此疾病的英国医生詹姆斯·帕金森的名字命名的）。

7. Étienne-Louis-Arthur Fallot (1850—1911)，法国内科学及病理学家，因其全面描述了法洛四联症的解剖学特征而载入医学史册。

Exercises

Ⅰ. **For each of the following statements, write "T" if the statement is true and "F" if the statement is false in the blank.**

_____ 1. Myocardial infarction refers to the necrosis of the coronary arteries.

_____ 2. Both angina and congestive heart failure are caused by an insufficient blood supply to the heart.

_____ 3. Vegetation of the heart valves may occur as a result of endocarditis.

_____ 4. Rheumatic heart disease mostly affects adults.

_____ 5. The weak points of artery walls are more susceptible to aneurysm.

_____ 6. No recognizable cause can be found for essential hypertension.

_____ 7. In patients with coarctation of the aorta, narrowing of the aorta results in increased blood pressure in the upper and lower extremities.

_____ 8. Surgery is found to be a common treatment for congenital heart diseases.

_____ 9. Atrial fibrillation is caused by the failure of an impulse to activate AV node.

_____ 10. Angina can result not only from abnormal heart rhythm but also from atherosclerosis.

Ⅱ. **Match each term in Column A with its correct description in Column B. Write the corresponding letter in the blank.**

Column A	Column B
_____ 1. pericardiocentesis	A. extremely rapid, incomplete contraction of muscle
_____ 2. aneurysm	B. bluish discoloration of the skin
_____ 3. implantation	C. situated or put under the skin
_____ 4. hypertrophy	D. arterial dilatation caused by weakening of vessel wall
_____ 5. fibrillation	E. a procedure to drain fluid from the pericardium
_____ 6. stenosis	F. an abnormal rate of muscle contractions in the heart
_____ 7. angioplasty	G. abnormal narrowing of a bodily canal or passageway
_____ 8. subcutaneous	H. a surgical procedure to place something in the body
_____ 9. arrhythmia	I. an operation to repair a damaged blood vessel
_____ 10. cyanosis	J. abnormal enlargement of a body part or organ

Ⅲ. **Translate the following Chinese sentences into English.**

1. 随着硬化的斑块在动脉内积聚，原光滑的血管壁变得粗糙。

2. 心绞痛常常因心肌供氧需求的增长而引发，比如在用力或压力状况下。

3. 心内膜炎指心脏瓣膜或腔室膜的感染，通常由细菌或其他微生物的直接侵入引发，会导致瓣膜尖变形。

4. 继发性高血压常伴有身体其他部位损伤，如肾小球性肾炎或肾上腺疾病，这些疾病往往引起血压升高。

5. 为了恢复正常的心跳节律，可在胸部安装一种叫作除颤器的电子装置，以矫正异常的心跳节律。

Ⅳ. Think critically and then answer the following questions.

1. Mr. Liu came to the hospital, presenting with the symptoms of weakness, fatigue, and an intermittent fever that persisted for weeks. The doctor ordered an echocardiogram for him and the result indicated vegetation on his mitral valve. What diagnosis would the doctor make?

2. A 45-year-old woman recently experienced episodes of severe pain in her left chest, sometimes radiating to the left shoulder and down the left arm. The pain usually occurred when she exerted herself to do housework or physical exercises, and disappeared after several minutes' rest. What would be the most likely cause of her chest pain?

Medicine in China

Tai Chi Good for Your Heart

People with heart disease, high blood pressure, or stroke may benefit from practicing traditional Chinese exercises such as Tai Chi, according to a study published in the *Journal of the American Heart Association*.

"Traditional Chinese exercises are a low-risk, promising intervention that can be helpful in improving quality of life in patients with cardiovascular diseases—the leading cause of disability and death in the world," the lead author Yu Liu, dean of the School of Kinesiology at Shanghai University of Sport in China, said.

In the new study, the researchers reviewed 35 research articles, which included 2,249 cardiovascular disease patients from 10 countries. They found that Chinese exercises helped reduce the participants' systolic blood pressure by more than 9.12 mm Hg, and diastolic blood pressure by more than 5 mm Hg on average. The study also revealed small, but statistically significant drops in the levels of bad cholesterol, or low-density lipoprotein, and triglycerides.

Chinese exercises also seemed to improve quality of life and reduce depression in patients with cardiovascular disease. "Our systematic review results showed that traditional Chinese exercises should be useful for patients with cardiovascular diseases," the researchers wrote in their paper.

The review analyzed studies which randomly assigned participants to groups performing traditional Chinese exercises, most commonly Tai Chi, Qigong, and Baduanjin, engaging in another form of exercise or making no change in activity level.

Exercises

Ⅰ. **Translate the underlined part into Chinese.**

Ⅱ. **Answer the following question.**

In what way can our heart benefit from traditional Chinese exercises?

Chapter 8

Respiratory System

Pre-Reading Question

What is Adam's apple? Is Adam's apple exclusively possessed by men?

Reading

Text A   Structure and Functions of the Respiratory System

The respiratory system is crucial to every human being. It serves the body much as a **lifeline** to an oxygen tank serves a **scuba** diver. Think how panicked you would feel if suddenly your lifeline became blocked and you could not breathe for a few seconds![1] A person can live a few weeks without food, a few days without water, but only a few minutes without oxygen.

The main function of the respiratory system is to supply life-sustaining oxygen to the body's cells and to remove from them, a waste product called carbon **dioxide**.[2] Breathing, or respiration, allows this important function to take place. Air carrying oxygen enters the body during **inhalation**, and air carrying carbon dioxide is **expelled** out of the body through **exhalation**. This exchange of gases is how the respiratory system helps maintain a constant environment that enables our body cells to function effectively.[3]

The process of breathing involves the proper functioning of various parts of the respiratory system. This body system can be divided into two sections—the upper and lower respiratory tracts. The upper section comprises the nose, pharynx (throat), and **larynx**. The lower respiratory tract is composed of the **trachea** or windpipe, bronchi, and lungs. Inside the lungs, each **bronchus** branches into **bronchioles** that end in millions of extremely tiny, very thin-walled sacs called **alveoli**. Figure 8-1 shows the extensive branching system of airway passages. This air distribution system may be considered as an "upside-down tree." The trachea then becomes the trunk and the **bronchial** tubes the branches.[4]

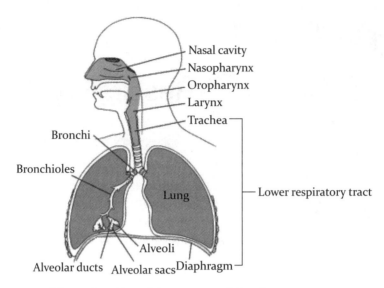

Figure 8-1   Branching system of the airway passage

The lungs are enclosed within the thoracic cavity. Thus changes in the shape and size of the thoracic cavity result in changes in the air pressure within that cavity and in the lungs. This difference in air pressure moves air from an area where pressure is high to an area where pressure is lower, causing the movement of air into and out of the lungs.[5] **Inspiratory** muscles, including the diaphragm and the external intercostals, are responsible for the increase in the volume of the thoracic cavity during **inspiration** or inhalation. The diaphragm is a sheet of muscles that lie beneath the lungs while the external intercostal muscles are located between the ribs. When the diaphragm contracts, it moves down toward the abdominal cavity, making the chest cavity longer from top to bottom. When the external intercostal muscles contract, they enlarge the thorax by increasing the size of the cavity from front to back and from side to side. **Contraction** of the inspiratory muscles increases the volume of the thoracic cavity and reduces lung air pressure below **atmospheric** air pressure, pulling air into the lungs. When the inspiratory muscles relax, the thoracic volume is reduced and the **intrapulmonary** pressure is increased, pumping air out of the lungs. This quiet, resting **expiration** or exhalation is a passive process, as it requires no muscular contraction. When we speak, sing, or do heavy work, we may need more forceful expiration to increase the rate and depth of ventilation. During forced expiration, the **expiratory** muscles (internal intercostals and abdominal muscles) contract to help push air out of the lungs. When contracted, the internal intercostal muscles pull the rib cage inward and decrease the front-to-back size of the thorax. Contraction of the abdominal muscles compresses the abdominal organs and pushes up on the diaphragm, and that further decreases the thoracic volume, increasing thoracic pressure and pushing the air out.

Alveoli[6] are where the exchange of oxygen and carbon dioxide takes place. These spongy, air-filled sacs are surrounded by capillaries. The **inhaled** oxygen passes into the alveoli and then **diffuses** through the capillaries into the arterial blood. Meanwhile, the waste-rich blood from the veins releases its carbon dioxide into the alveoli. The carbon dioxide follows the same path out of the lungs when one **exhales**. Two structural characteristics of the alveoli facilitate gas exchange. First, the wall of each alveolus is made up of a single layer of cells and so are the walls of the capillaries around it.[7] This means that there is a barrier probably less than 1 **micron** thick between the blood in the capillaries and the air in the alveolus. This extremely thin barrier is called the respiratory membrane. Second, there are millions of alveoli and together they make an enormous surface area (an area many times larger than the surface of the entire body) for quick gas exchange.

Respiratory **mucosa** is the membrane lining the respiratory tract, including the **nasal** cavity, larynx, trachea, and bronchial tree. Respiratory mucosa consists of a **pseudo-stratified columnar** epithelium with **cilia** and **goblet** cells and is covered with a layer of protective mucus, which serves as the most important air **purification** mechanism. Only the **vocal** cords are free of this **mucous** coating. More than 125 mL of respiratory mucus is produced daily. Air is **purified** when **contaminants** such as dust, **pollen**, and bacterial organisms stick to the mucus and become trapped. Normally, the mucus containing inhaled contaminants moves upward from the lower portions of the bronchial tree on the millions of hairlike cilia that beat or move only in one direction. When the debris-filled mucus reaches the pharynx, it is usually swallowed and travels to the acid environment of the stomach.

▶ Word Bank

lifeline /'laɪflaɪn/ *n.* 救生索；生命线

scuba /'sku:bə/ *n.* 水中呼吸器

dioxide /daɪ'ɒksaɪd/ *n.* 二氧化物

inhalation /ˌɪnhə'leɪʃən/ *n.* 吸入

expel /ɪk'spel/ *v.* 驱逐；排出

exhalation /ˌekshə'leɪʃən/ *n.* 呼气

larynx /'lærɪŋks/　 *n.* 喉

trachea /'treɪkɪə/ *n.* 气管

bronchus /'brɒŋkəs/ *n.* 支气管（复数为 bronchi）

bronchiole /'brɒŋkɪəʊl/ *n.* 细支气管，小支气管

alveolus /'ælvɪ·ələs/ *n.* 肺泡；小窝（复数为 alveoli）

bronchial /'brɒŋkɪəl/ *a.* 支气管的

inspiratory /ɪn'spaɪrətərɪ/ *a.* 吸入的；吸气的

inspiration /ˌɪnspɪ'reɪʃən/ *n.* 吸气

contraction /kən'trækʃən/ *n.* 收缩

atmospheric /ˌætməs'ferɪk/ *a.* 大气的，大气层的

intrapulmonary /ˌɪntrə'pʌlmənərɪ/ *a.* 肺内的

expiration /ˌekspɪ'reɪʃən/ *n.* 呼气

expiratory /eks'paɪrətərɪ/ *a.* 呼气的

inhale /ɪn'heɪl/ *v.* 吸入

diffuse /dɪ'fju:z/ *v.* 扩散；传播

exhale /ɪks'heɪl/ *v.* 呼气

micron /'maɪkrɒn/ *n.* 微米（等于百万分之一米）

mucosa /mju:'kəʊsə/ *n.* 黏膜

nasal /'neɪzəl/ *a.* 鼻的

pseudo-stratified /'sju:dəʊ'strætɪfaɪd/ *a.* 假复层的

columnar /kə'lʌmnə/ *a.* 柱状的

cilium /'sɪlɪəm/ *n.* 纤毛（复数为 cilia）

goblet /'gɒblɪt/ *n.* 酒杯；高脚杯

vocal /'vəʊkəl/ *a.* 声音的

purify /'pjʊrɪfaɪ/ *v.* 使纯净；去除

pollen /'pɒlən/ *n.* 花粉

purification /ˌpjʊərɪfɪ'keɪʃən/ *n.* 净化；提纯

mucous /'mjuːkəs/ *a.* 黏液的；分泌黏液的

contaminant /kən'tæmɪnənt/ *n.* 污染物；污垢物

▶ Notes

1. 该句为虚拟条件句。虚拟条件句往往描述不能实现或纯假想的情况，可以对过去、现在或将来进行假想。本句为对现在的假设。if 引导的条件句用一般过去时态（became blocked 和 could not breathe），主句用 would/could/should/might do something (would feel panicked)。

2. 不定式短语 to supply life-sustaining oxygen to the body's cells and to remove from them, a waste product called carbon dioxide 在句中作表语。a waste product called carbon dioxide 是 remove 的宾语，called carbon dioxide 为过去分词短语，作 a waste product 的定语。为了保持句子平衡，避免头重脚轻，remove 的宾语后置，放在句尾。

3. how the respiratory system helps maintain a constant environment that enables our body cells to function effectively 是表语从句。that enables our body cells to function effectively 为定语从句，修饰 a constant environment。这种从句套从句的复杂结构是医学英语语篇的一个特点。

4. 该句为并列句，and 连接的后半部分省略了动词 become。

5. where pressure is high 及 where pressure is lower 为定语从句，分别修饰它们各自前面的名词 an area。现在分词短语 causing the movement of air into and out of the lungs 在句中作结果状语。

6. alveoli 是 alveolus 的复数形式。以 -us 结尾的很多医学英语词汇都源于拉丁语，因而在变复数时遵循拉丁语的规则：变 -us 为 -i，又如：bronchus 的复数为 bronchi，fungus 的复数为 fungi。

7. so are the walls of the capillaries around it 为倒装句结构，相当于 the walls of the capillaries around it are made up of a single layer of cells as well。为了避免与前半部分的表语重复，该句中用 so 代替 made up of a single layer of cells，并将 so 及助动词 are 提到主语前。so + 助动词 / 情态动词 + 主语这一倒装结构表示前一情况的重复出现，常翻译为 "……也……"。

Exercises

Ⅰ. **Choose the best answer to each of the following questions.**

1. The _____ is part of the upper respiratory tract.
   A. lung   B. trachea
   C. bronchus   D. larynx

2. The bronchi are connected to the alveoli via _____.
   A. capillaries   B. air sacs
   C. bronchioles   D. the trachea

3. What surrounds each alveolar sac?
   A. Capillaries.   B. Veins.
   C. Arteries.   D. Lymphatic ducts.

4. Gas exchange in the lungs occurs between blood in the _____ and air in the _____.
   A. veins; bronchi   B. arteries; bronchioles
   C. lymphatic ducts; alveoli D. capillaries; alveoli

5. Air moves out of the lungs when the pressure inside the lungs is _____.
   A. less than the pressure in the atmosphere
   B. greater than the pressure in the atmosphere
   C. equal to the pressure in the atmosphere
   D. greater than the intra-alveolar pressure

6. When the external intercostal muscles and diaphragm contract, the thoracic cavity _____ and the air pressure in the lungs _____.
   A. expands; increases   B. contracts; decreases
   C. expands; decreases   D. contracts; increases

7. Blood flowing into lung capillaries has a higher concentration of _____, which is expelled out of the body through _____.
   A. oxygen; inhalation   B. carbon dioxide; exhalation
   C. water; inhalation   D. fluid; exhalation

8. What is the main function of the cilia hairs and mucus of the conducting passages?
   A. To speed up gas exchange in the alveoli.
   B. To lower the air pressure in the lungs.
   C. To reduce the alveolar surface tension.
   D. To filter impurities from the inhaled air.

9. The diffusion of alveolar oxygen into the blood is rapid and involves diffusion across _____ layers of cells.

    A. 5   B. 4   C. 3   D. 2

10. What happens to the mucus that is pushed to the top of the respiratory tract?

    A. It is swallowed.   B. It is broken down.

    C. It is stored.   D. It is absorbed.

Ⅱ. **Write the names of the respiratory system structures in the spaces given.**

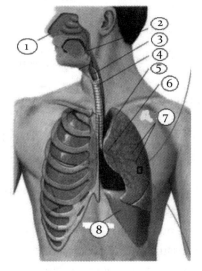

1. _____   2. _____

3. _____   4. _____

5. _____   6. _____

7. _____   8. _____

Ⅲ. **Fill in each blank in the following paragraph with a word in the box. Change the form of words if necessary.**

mucus	pollution	bronchial	infection	pollutant
result	mechanism	cilium	digest	inhalation
particle	lining	pulmonary	bronchitis	swallow

The lungs have several ways of protecting themselves from irritants. First, the nose acts as a filter during 1_____, preventing large particles of

2 _____ from entering the lungs. If an irritant does enter the lung, it will get stuck in a thin layer of mucus secreted onto the 3 _____ of the breathing tubes. This mucus is "swept up" by little hairs called 4 _____ toward the mouth, where the mucus is 5 _____. Spitting up sputum（痰）does not occur unless the individual has chronic 6 _____ or there is a(n) 7 _____ such as a chest cold or pneumonia. Another protective 8 _____ for the lungs is the cough. A cough is the result of irritation to the 9 _____ tubes. A cough can expel 10 _____ from the lungs faster than cilia.

Ⅳ. **Translate the following English sentences into Chinese.**

1. How panicked you would feel if suddenly your lifeline became blocked and you could not breathe for a few seconds!

2. This exchange of gases is how the respiratory system helps maintain a constant environment that enables our body cells to function effectively.

3. This difference in air pressure moves air from an area where pressure is high to an area where pressure is lower, causing the movement of air into and out of the lungs.

4. Contraction of the abdominal muscles compresses the abdominal organs and pushes up on the diaphragm, and that further decreases the thoracic volume, increasing thoracic pressure and pushing the air out.

5. Normally, the mucus containing inhaled contaminants moves upward from the lower portions of the bronchial tree on the millions of hairlike cilia that beat or move only in one direction.

Ⅳ. **Write a 100-word summary of the gas exchange in the lungs.**

Reading

Text B Diseases of the Respiratory System and Their Treatment

Respiratory diseases are among the ten leading causes of death in China. They affect the respiratory system including the upper respiratory tract, trachea, bronchi, bronchioles, alveoli, **pleura** and **pleural** cavity, and the nerves and muscles of breathing. Respiratory diseases range from mild and **self-limiting**, such as the common cold, to life-threatening **entities** like bacterial **pneumonia**, pulmonary

embolism, and lung cancer.

Respiratory Tract Infections

Respiratory tract infections are caused by bacteria, viruses or even fungi. Infections can affect any part of the respiratory system and are traditionally divided into upper respiratory tract infections and lower respiratory tract infections. The most common upper respiratory tract infection is the common cold. However, infections of specific organs of the upper respiratory tract such as **sinusitis**, **tonsillitis**, **otitis** media, **pharyngitis**, and **laryngitis** are also considered upper respiratory tract infections. Lower respiratory tract infections affect the trachea or windpipe and lungs and include **bronchitis** (infection of the large airways or bronchi), **bronchiolitis** (infection of the small airways or bronchioles), **emphysema**, **asthma**, **croup** (infection of the trachea or windpipe in children), and pneumonia.

The flu is a **viral** infection of the upper and lower respiratory tracts, including the nose, throat and, occasionally, bronchi and lungs. The flu is characterized by chills, fever, headache, and muscular aches, in addition to respiratory symptoms. There are several strains of flu viruses. The mortality rate of the flu is approximately 1%, and most of those deaths are among the very old and very young. During a flu **epidemic** the infection rate is so rapid and the disease is so widespread that the total number of deaths is substantial, even though the percentage of deaths is relatively low. Flu **vaccines** can provide protection against the flu.

The most common lower respiratory tract infection is pneumonia, an infection of the alveoli and surrounding lung tissue. Many **germs**, such as bacteria, viruses, and fungi, can cause pneumonia. You can also get pneumonia by inhaling a liquid or chemical. People most at risk are those who are older than 65 or younger than 2 years of age, or already have health problems. Symptoms include fever, difficulty in breathing, and chest pain. Inflammation of the lungs results in the accumulation of fluid within alveoli (pulmonary edema) and poor **inflation** of the lungs with air. A **protozoal** infection that results in **pneumocystosis** pneumonia is rare, except in persons who have a **compromised** immune system. This type of pneumonia has become one of the infections commonly suffered by persons with AIDS.

Chronic Obstructive Pulmonary Disorders

Common chronic obstructive pulmonary disorders (COPDs) include asthma, chronic bronchitis, and emphysema. Asthma is a disorder in which there are **periodic episodes** of contractions of bronchial smooth muscle, which restricts air movement. Many cases of asthma result from **allergic** responses to pollen, dust, animal **dander**, or other substances. Treatment includes the use of drugs that relax the bronchiole smooth muscles and reduce inflammation. Sometimes injections are given to reduce the sensitivity of the immune system to the substances that stimulate an asthma attack.

Bronchitis is an inflammation of the bronchi caused by irritants, such as cigarette smoke, air pollution, or infections. The inflammation results in swelling of the mucous membrane lining the bronchi, increased mucus production, and decreased movement of mucus by cilia.[1] Consequently, the diameter of the bronchi is decreased and ventilation is impaired.

Bronchitis can progress to emphysema. Narrowing of the bronchioles restricts air movement, and air tends to be **retained** in the lungs. Coughing to remove accumulated mucus increases pressure in the alveoli, resulting in rupture and destruction of **alveolar** walls and the occurrence of emphysema. Loss of alveolar walls has two important consequences. The respiratory membrane has a decreased surface area, which decreases gas exchange, and the loss of elastic fibers decreases the ability of the lungs to **recoil** and expel air. Symptoms of emphysema include shortness of breath and enlargement of the thoracic cavity. Treatment involves removing sources of irritants (for example, stopping smoking), promoting the removal of bronchial secretions, retraining people to breathe so that expiration of air is **maximized**, and using antibiotics to prevent infections. The progress of emphysema can be slowed, but there is no cure.

Tuberculosis

Tuberculosis is caused by a tuberculosis bacterium. In the lung, the tuberculosis bacteria form lesions called **tubercles**. The small lumps contain **degenerating macrophages** and tuberculosis bacteria. An immune reaction is directed against the tubercles, which causes the formation of larger lesions and inflammation. The tubercles can rupture, releasing bacteria that infect other parts of the lung or body. Recently, a strain of drug-resistant tuberculosis bacteria has developed, and there is concern that tuberculosis will again become a widespread infectious disease.

Pulmonary Fibrosis

Pulmonary fibrosis, a disease marked by **scarring** in the lungs, is the formation or development of excess fibrous connective tissue in the lungs. Pulmonary fibrosis is suggested by a history of progressive shortness of breath (**dyspnea**[2]) with exertion. Sometimes fine inspiratory **crackles** can be heard at the lung bases on[3] **auscultation**. A chest X-ray may or may not be abnormal, but high-**resolution** CT will frequently demonstrate abnormalities. Exposure to **asbestos**, **silica**, or coal dust is the most common cause. However, most cases of pulmonary fibrosis have no known cause. These cases are called idiopathic pulmonary fibrosis. Pulmonary fibrosis can develop slowly or quickly. There is no cure and current treatments for pulmonary fibrosis cannot remove scarring that has already occurred. Many people with the disease live only about three to five years after diagnosis.

Lung Cancer

Lung cancer arises from the epithelium of the respiratory tract. Cancers arising from tissues other than respiratory epithelium are not called lung cancer, even though they occur in the lungs. Lung cancer is the most common cause of cancer death in males and females in the United States and China, and almost all cases occur in smokers. Because of the rich **lymph** and blood supply in the lungs, cancer in the lung can readily spread to other parts of the lung or body. In addition, the disease is often **advanced**[4] before symptoms become severe enough for the victim to seek medical aid. Typical symptoms include coughing, **sputum** production, and blockage of the airways. Treatments include removal of part or all of the lung, chemotherapy, and radiation.

▶ Word Bank

pleura /'plʊərə/ *n.* 胸膜；肋膜

pleural /'plʊərəl/ *a.* 胸膜的；肋膜的

self-limiting /self'lɪmɪtɪŋ/ *a.* 自限性的

entity /'entɪtɪ/ *n.* 病种，疾病

pneumonia /nju:'məʊnɪə/ *n.* 肺炎

embolism /'embə‚lɪzəm/ *n.* 栓塞

sinusitis /‚saɪnə'saɪtɪs/ *n.* 鼻窦炎

tonsillitis /‚tɒnsɪ'laɪtɪs/ *n.* 扁桃腺炎

otitis /əʊ'taɪtɪs/ *n.* 耳炎

pharyngitis /‚færɪn'dʒaɪtɪs/ *n.* 咽炎

laryngitis /‚lærɪn'dʒaɪtɪs/ *n.* 喉炎

bronchitis /brɒŋ'kaɪtɪs/ *n.* 支气管炎

bronchiolitis /‚brɒŋkɪəʊ'laɪtɪs/ *n.* 细支气管炎

emphysema /‚emfɪ'si:mə/ *n.* 气肿；肺气肿

asthma /'æsmə/ *n.* 哮喘

croup /kru:p/ *n.* 哮吼

viral /'vaɪrəl/ *a.* 病毒性的

epidemic /‚epɪ'demɪk/ *n.* 传染病；流行病

vaccine /'væksi:n/ *n.* 疫苗

germ /dʒɜ:m/ *n.* 细菌；病菌

inflation /ɪn'fleɪʃən/ *n.* 膨胀

protozoal /‚prəʊtəʊ'zəʊəl/ *a.* 原生动物的

pneumocystosis /‚nju:məsɪs'təʊsɪs/ *n.* 肺孢子虫病

compromised /'kɒmprəmaɪzd/ *a.* 缺乏抵抗力的

obstructive /əb'strʌktɪv/ *a.* 阻塞性的；妨碍的

periodic /‚pɪərɪ'ɒdɪk/ *a.* 周期的；定期的

episode /'epɪsəʊd/ *n.* 发作

allergic /ə'lɜ:dʒɪk/ *a.* 对……过敏的

dander /'dændə/ *n.* 头皮屑

retain /rɪ'teɪn/ *v.* 保留，保存

alveolar /æl'vɪələ/ *a.* 肺泡的

recoil /rɪ'kɒɪl/ *v.* 弹回

maximize /'mæksɪmaɪz/ *v.* 最大化

tubercle /'tju:bɜ:kl/ *n.* 结节

degenerate /dɪ'dʒenəreɪt/ *v.* 使退化；恶化

macrophage /'mækrəʊfeɪdʒ/ *n.* 巨噬细胞

scarring /'skɑ:rɪŋ/ *n.* 瘢痕形成

dyspnea /dɪs'pni:ə/ *n.* 呼吸困难

crackle /'krækl/ *n.* 爆裂声

resolution /ˌrezə'luːʃən/ *n.* 清晰度；分辨率

silica /'sɪlɪkə/ *n.* 二氧化硅

advanced /əd'vɑːnst/ *a.* 晚期的

auscultation /ˌɔːskəl'teɪʃən/ *n.* 听诊

asbestos /æs'bestəs/ *n.* 石棉

lymph /lɪmf/ *n.* 淋巴液

sputum /'spjuːtəm/ *n.* 痰

▶ Notes

1. 该句中过去分词 increased 和 decreased 为定语，分别修饰名词短语 mucus production 和 movement of mucus by cilia。lining the bronchi 为现在分词充当定语修饰 the mucous membrane。increased mucus production，decreased movement of mucus by cilia 与 swelling of the mucous membrane lining the bronchi 为名词短语，共同充当短语动词 result in 的宾语。by cilia 为定语修饰 movement。

2. dyspnea 呼吸困难。此词由前缀 dys-（困难）和词根 -pnea（呼吸）构成。dys-还有异常之意。例如：dysfunction（功能异常）。

3. 该句中介词 on 表示当……的时候，例如：No abnormal behavior was found on examination.（检查时未发现行为异常。）。

4. advanced 在此处是医学词汇，意为晚期的。

Exercises

Ⅰ. **For each of the following statements, write "T" if the statement is true and "F" if the statement is false in the blank.**

_____ 1. The common cold is an upper respiratory tract infection while the flu is a lower respiratory tract infection.

_____ 2. Pneumonia is caused by inhalation of a liquid or chemical.

_____ 3. People with AIDS are often vulnerable to pneumocystosis pneumonia.

_____ 4. During an asthma attack, the bronchioles dilate.

_____ 5. Emphysema results in permanent damage to the alveoli.

_____ 6. The lungs contract to force the air out of the lungs.

_____ 7. At present severe emphysema is curable.

_____ 8. Inhaling particles such as silica and coal dust can lead to pulmonary fibrosis.

_____ 9. Dyspnea is a medical term for chest pain.

_____ 10. Lung cancer is strongly correlated with cigarette smoking.

Ⅱ. **Match each term in Column A with its correct description in Column B. Write the corresponding letter in the blank.**

Column A	Column B
_____ 1. pharyngitis	A. swelling from excessive accumulation of watery fluid in cells, tissues, or serous cavities
_____ 2. tubercle	B. an obstructive disorder characterized by recurring spasms of the smooth muscles of the bronchi
_____ 3. pulmonary embolism	C. an inflammation or infection of the pharynx
_____ 4. asthma	D. an inflammation of the larynx
_____ 5. laryngitis	E. a swelling that is the characteristic lesion of tuberculosis
_____ 6. auscultation	F. development of excess fibrous connective tissue in an organ
_____ 7. emphysema	G. blockage of the pulmonary artery by foreign matter or by a blood clot
_____ 8. edema	H. an acute inflammation of the lungs
_____ 9. pneumonia	I. a condition in which ruptured alveoli reduce the surface area of the lung, making breathing difficult
_____ 10. fibrosis	J. listening to sounds within the body usually with a stethoscope

Ⅲ. **Translate the following Chinese sentences into English.**

1. 呼吸系统疾病包括从轻度的自限性疾病（如普通感冒）到威胁生命的细菌性肺炎、肺栓塞和肺癌等疾病。

2. 年龄超过 65 岁或小于 2 岁，或者已经存在健康问题的人群最易感染肺炎。

3. 患哮喘时，支气管平滑肌会周期性收缩，限制空气流动。

4. 炎症可导致支气管黏膜肿胀，黏液产生增多，并且纤毛带动的黏液运动减少。

5. 不是起源于呼吸道上皮组织的癌症，即使它们出现在肺部，也不称之为肺癌。

Ⅳ. **Think critically and then answer the following questions.**

1. Why are children who attend day-care centers more likely to contract pneumonia than kids who stay at home?

2. Mr. Johnson came to the clinic complaining of dyspnea. What lung disease(s) might he suffer from? List the possible lung diseases he might suffer from.

Medicine in China

TCM Effective in Treating Respiratory Diseases and Cancer

Chinese medical experts have highlighted the role of Traditional Chinese Medicine (TCM) in treating respiratory and lung diseases, as well as cancer.

Zhang Hongchun, head of the TCM Department at China-Japan Friendship Hospital, said their TCM prescriptions have proven effective in treating infectious respiratory symptoms, such as relieving and shortening symptoms of flu patients and alleviating coughing of COVID-19 patients in recovery.

Because it takes time for scientists to develop vaccines and targeted Western medications for infectious illnesses, Zhang said that TCM specialists are able to promptly formulate prescriptions by observing and analyzing the condition of patients. Rather than fighting off viruses, TCM mainly focuses on regulating the condition of the body, reducing inflammatory reactions, and minimizing damage to organs. Regarding interstitial lung diseases—illnesses that cause scarring of the lungs, Zhang said TCM medicines can help lower the dosage of hormone, alleviate side effects of hormone, and enhance the immunity of patients.

Jia Liqun, head of the hospital's Oncology Department of Integrated TCM and Western Medicine, said that TCM therapies, when combined with Western Medicine, can play a role in tackling precancerous lesions, alleviating adverse reactions of Western drugs, and improving life quality of late-stage cancer patients.

Exercises

Ⅰ. **Translate the underlined part into Chinese.**

Ⅱ. **Answer the following question.**

How can TCM treat respiratory diseases effectively?

Chapter 9

Nervous System ◀

Pre-Reading Question

What is the meaning of "An idle brain is the devil's workshop"? What do you think those people with "idle brain" are likely to do?

Reading

Text A Structure and Functions of the Nervous System

The nervous system is essentially a biological information highway and is responsible for controlling all the biological processes and movements in the body. It consists of the central nervous system (CNS), essentially the processing area, and the **peripheral** nervous system (PNS) which detects and sends electrical impulses used in the nervous system. The CNS, the center of the nervous system, consists of the brain and spinal cord (Figure 9-1).

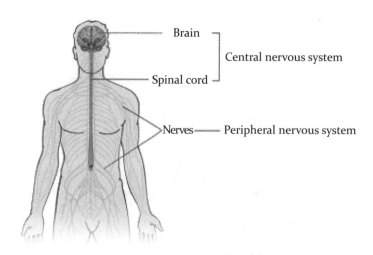

Figure 9-1   Structure of the nervous system

The brain has a **jelly**-like consistency, containing one hundred billion neurons, and weighs around 1.5 kilograms, which allows us to feel emotions and carry out our thought processes. This primary control center is divided into the **brainstem**, **cerebellum**, and **cerebrum**.

The brainstem is the connection between the brain and the rest of the CNS. This is commonly referred to as[1] the simplest part of the brain, as most creatures on the evolutionary scale have some form of brain creation that resembles the brain stem. In humans, this area contains the **medulla, midbrain**, and **pons**. The midbrain, also known as the **mesencephalon**, is made up of the **tegmentum** and **tectum**. These parts of the brain help regulate body movement, vision, and hearing. The pons are located in the **hindbrain** and link to the cerebellum to help with posture and movement. The pons also create the level of consciousness necessary for sleep. The medulla or medulla **oblongata** maintains vital body functions such as heart rate and breathing.

The cerebellum is found below the **occipital** lobe and adjacent to the brainstem. The cerebellum is primarily responsible for controlling movement, helping the body operate in balance and **equilibrium**, and transmitting sensory information.

The cerebrum is the largest part of the human brain and lies above the brainstem and cerebellum. This part is responsible for intelligence and creativity and is also involved in memory. The "grey matter" of the cerebrum is the cerebral cortex, dealing with almost all of the higher functions of an intelligent being. It is this part that translates our nervous impulses into understandable **quantifiable** feelings and thoughts.[2]

The cerebral cortex is divided into four sections: the temporal lobe, the occipital lobe, the parietal lobe, and the **frontal** lobe. The frontal lobe is found at the front of the head, near the **temple** and forehead. It is essential to many of the advanced functions of an evolved brain, including creative thought, problem solving, **intellect**, judgment, attention, abstract thinking, physical reactions, smell, and personality. The parietal lobe is situated behind the frontal lobe, receiving information **relayed** from the spinal cord regarding the position of various body parts, and monitoring and controlling movement throughout the body. The temporal lobe is located in parallel with[3] the ears. It serves the ears by interpreting audio signals received from the **auditory** canal. The occipital lobe, the smallest of the four lobe components of the cerebrum, is located at the back of the brain and is responsible for interpreting nerve signals from the eye.

The **limbic** system of the cerebrum contains glands which help relay emotions. Many hormonal responses that the body generates are initiated in this area.

The limbic system includes the **amygdala**, hippocampus, **hypothalamus**, and **thalamus**. The amygdala helps the body respond to emotions, memories, and fear. It is a large portion of the **telencephalon**, located within the temporal lobe which can be seen from the surface of the brain. The hypothalamus, about the size of a pearl, directs a **multitude** of important functions. It wakes you up in the morning and gets the **adrenaline** flowing[4] during a test or job interview. The hypothalamus, also an important emotional center, controls the molecules that make you feel **exhilarated**, angry, or unhappy. Near the hypothalamus lies the thalamus, a major **clearinghouse** for information going to and from the spinal cord and the cerebrum. An **arching** tract of nerve cells leads from the hypothalamus and the thalamus to the hippocampus. This tiny **nub** acts as a memory **indexer**—sending memories out to the appropriate part of the cerebral **hemisphere** for long-term storage and **retrieving** them when necessary. The **basal ganglia** are **clusters** of nerve cells surrounding the thalamus. They are responsible for initiating and **integrating** movements.

The spinal cord is a long, white tube made up of support cells and nerve tissues, extending downwards from the medulla oblongata. The spinal cord is responsible for three main functions: carrying information, coordinating **reflexes**, and controlling reflexes. The spinal cord delivers information to and from the brain. Information from the sensory receptors in the body is taken to the spinal cord **via** the **afferent** nerves, which is then sent along to the brain, and information from the brain is delivered to different muscles and glands in the body via **efferent** fibers. The spinal cord is also capable of coordinating reflexes on its own and is, therefore, responsible for **integrative** functions and communications. The spinal cord controls reflex actions. Reflex actions are those actions that are sudden, involuntary, and automatic response actions, typically exhibited by humans when the survival instinct kicks in or when danger is detected.

The **autonomic** nervous system is a part of the peripheral nervous system and is also known as the **visceral** nervous system or involuntary nervous system. It forms one of the many control systems of the body and does not operate at the full level of consciousness. It is divided into the **sympathetic** nervous system and the **parasympathetic** nervous system. The sympathetic nervous system activates the fight or flight mechanism in a human when he or she detects danger or is threatened. In this state, a redirection of energy takes place; digestion is put on hold[5], **pupils dilate**, heart rate and breathing rate **escalate**, and there is increased production of **saliva** and sweat. The parasympathetic nervous system has the opposite effect on the organs.

The somatic nervous system is a part of the peripheral nervous system and is also known as the voluntary nervous system. It is involved in the control and regulation of voluntary movements via the skeletal muscles and contains efferent nerves, which are associated with muscle contraction. The somatic nervous system consists of spinal nerves, **cranial** nerves, and association nerves. Spinal nerves are responsible for the transmission of sensory information into the spinal cord. Cranial nerves are responsible for conducting information, such as smell, vision, and taste, to and from the brain stem. Association nerves are responsible for associating and coordinating motor output with the sensory input received.

The CNS receives and interprets signals from the peripheral nervous system and also sends out signals to it, either consciously or unconsciously. This information highway consists of many nerve cells, also known as neurons, as seen below.

Each neuron consists of a nucleus situated in the cell body, from which **outgrowths** called **processes**[6] originate. The largest one of these processes is the **axon**, which is responsible for carrying outgoing messages from the cell. **Dendrites** are smaller secondary processes that grow from the cell body. On the end of the axon lie the axon **terminals**, which "plug" into a cell where the electrical signal from a nerve cell to the target cell can be made. This "plug" (the axon terminal) connects to a receptor on the target cell and can transmit information between cells.

The neuron is usually surrounded by many support cells. Some types of cells wrap around the axon to form an insulating **sheath**. This sheath can include a fatty molecule called **myelin**, which provides insulation for the axon and helps nerve signals travel faster and farther. When the signal reaches the end of the axon, it stimulates the release of tiny sacs. These sacs release chemicals known as **neurotransmitters** into the **synapse**. The neurotransmitters cross the synapse and attach to receptors on the neighboring cell.

The nervous system is **inarguably** the most important part of the body because of the way it controls the biological processes of our body and all conscious thoughts. Due to its importance, it is safely **encased** within bones, namely, the cranium protecting the brain and the spine protecting the spinal cord.

▶ Word Bank

peripheral /pə'rɪfərəl/ *a.* 外围的，外周的

brainstem /'breɪnstem/ *n.* 脑干

cerebrum /sə'ri:brəm/ *n.* 大脑

midbrain /'mɪdbreɪn/ *n.* 中脑

mesencephalon /ˌmesen'sefəlɒn/ *n.* 中脑

tectum /'tektəm/ *n.* 顶盖

oblongata /ˌɒblɒŋ'ga:tə/ *n.* 延髓

jelly /'dʒelɪ/ *n.* 果冻；胶状物

cerebellum /ˌserə'beləm/ *n.* 小脑

medulla /mɪ'dju:lə/ *n.* 髓质，骨髓

pons /pɒnz/ *n.* 脑桥

tegmentum /teg'mentəm/ *n.* 被盖

hindbrain /'haɪndbreɪn/ *n.* 后脑

occipital /ɒk'sɪpɪtəl/ *a.* 枕骨的

equilibrium /ˌi:kwɪˈlɪbrɪəm/ *n.* 平衡，均衡

frontal /ˈfrʌntəl/ *a.* 前的，额的

intellect /ˈɪntəlekt/ *n.* 智力

auditory /ˈɔːdətərɪ/ *a.* 听觉的

amygdala /əˈmɪgdələ/ *n.* 杏仁核

thalamus /ˈθæləməs/ *n.* 丘脑

multitude /ˈmʌltɪtjuːd/ *n.* 大量

exhilarated /ɪgˈzɪləreɪtɪd/ *a.* 高兴的，愉快的

arching /ˈɑːtʃɪŋ/ *a.* 成拱形的

indexer /ˈɪndeksə/ *n.* 指针；指示器

retrieve /rɪˈtriːv/ *v.* 取回；检索

ganglion /ˈgæŋglɪən/ *n.* 神经节（复数为 ganglia）

integrate /ˈɪntɪgreɪt/ *v.* 整合，结合

via /vaɪə/ *prep.* 经由，通过

efferent /ˈefərənt/ *a.* 传出的

autonomic /ˌɔːtəˈnɒmɪk/ *a.* 自主的，自律的

sympathetic /ˌsɪmpəˈθetɪk/ *a.* 交感（神经）的

parasympathetic /ˌpærəˌsɪmpəˈθetɪk/ *a.* 副交感（神经）的

pupil /ˈpjuːpl/ *n.* 瞳孔

escalate /ˈeskəleɪt/ *v.* 加速

cranial /ˈkreɪnɪəl/ *a.* 颅的

process /ˈprəʊses/ *n.* 突起

dendrite /ˈdendraɪt/ *n.* 树突

sheath /ʃiːθ/ *n.* 髓鞘

neurotransmitter /ˌnjʊərəʊˈtrænzmɪtə/ *n.* 神经递质

inarguably /ɪnˈɑːgjʊəbəlɪ/ *ad.* 不容争辩地，没有疑问地

quantifiable /ˈkwɒntɪfaɪəbl/ *a.* 可量化的

temple /ˈtempl/ *n.* 太阳穴

relay /ˈriːleɪ/ *v.* 传递，转达

limbic /ˈlɪmbɪk/ *a.* （脑）边的，边缘的

hypothalamus /ˌhaɪpəˈθæləməs/ *n.* 下丘脑

telencephalon /ˌtelenˈsefəlɒn/ *n.* 端脑，终脑

adrenaline /əˈdrenəlɪn/ *n.* 肾上腺素

clearinghouse /ˈklɪrɪŋˌhaʊs/ *n.* 交换场所

nub /nʌb/ *n.* 小肿块

hemisphere /ˈhemɪsfɪə/ *n.* 半球

basal /ˈbeɪsəl/ *a.* 基底的

cluster /ˈklʌstə/ *n.* 群，簇

reflex /ˈriːfleks/ *n.* 反射

afferent /ˈæfərənt/ *a.* 传入的

integrative /ˈɪntɪgreɪtɪv/ *a.* 综合的，整合的

visceral /ˈvɪsərəl/ *a.* 内脏的

dilate /daɪˈleɪt/ *v.* 使扩大

saliva /səˈlaɪvə/ *n.* 唾液

outgrowth /ˈaʊtgrəʊθ/ *n.* 长出物

axon /ˈæksɒn/ *n.* 轴突

terminal /ˈtɜːmɪnəl/ *n.* 末端

myelin /ˈmaɪəlɪn/ *n.* 髓磷脂

synapse /ˈsaɪnæps/ *n.* 突触

encase /ɪnˈkeɪs/ *v.* 包起，裹起

▶ Notes

1. be referred to as 此词组常用来下定义，表示"被定义为……"，"被认为……"。如：Angina is often referred to as a symptom of coronary heart disease.（心绞痛常被认为是冠心病的一种症状。）。在医学文献中用来定义或解释术语的类似表达法有 be known as, be called, be defined as, be described as 等。

2. 该句为强调句，主语 this part（即 cerebral cortex）是被强调的部分，该句的原有结构是 This part translates our nervous impulses into understandable quantifiable feelings and thoughts.。强调句的构成为 It is (was) + 被强调部分 + that + 句子的其他成分，用以突出句中的主语、宾语和状语。如果被强调的主语是人，that 也可改用 who。

3. in parallel with 这个词组的意思为与……平行，和……同时。如：This decline in mental capacity is apparently in parallel with the advancing stages of Alzheimer's.

（智力能力的下降显然是与阿尔茨海默病病程同步发展的。）在医学文献中，以下词组也常用来表示组织器官的方位。如：anterior to 在……之前，posterior to 在……之后，adjacent to 与……相邻，perpendicular to 垂直于……，in proximity to 与……相近。

4. get the adrenaline flowing 这个词组的意思为使得肾上腺素水平升高。此词组已被借用到日常用语中，逐渐丧失了其原有的专业含义，可直接译为使兴奋，使热血沸腾。另外，get 是使役动词，相当于make 或have。get sth flowing 表示 "使充满……"，如 get your creative juice flowing 表示展开你丰富的创造想象力，get ideas flowing 表示使思想活跃。

5. put on hold 是个固定短语，表示搁置、延期、暂停。如：Anti-aging expert Barbara Morris explains in her book how to put the aging process on hold and stay youthful, dynamic, and healthy.（抗衰老专家芭芭拉·莫里斯在她的著作中阐述了如何延缓衰老，永葆青春、活力和健康。）

6. processes 在此处的意思不是过程、进程，而是突起。专业文献中常常会出现一些日常用词，但它们却具有不为学习者熟知的专业意义，切不可想当然地理解，一定要多查专业词典。例如，在医学中 colony 意为菌落，culture 意为（组织细胞的）培养，piles 意为痔疮，temple 意为太阳穴，tender 意为触痛，dress 意为敷药。

Exercises

Ⅰ. **Choose the best answer to each of the following questions.**

1. Which part of the brain maintains the heart rate and breathing function of the body?
   A. The midbrain.
   B. The medulla.
   C. The pons.
   D. The tegmentum.

2. The cerebellum is situated _____.
   A. above the brainstem
   B. below the medulla
   C. beside the temporal lobe
   D. below the occipital lobe

3. The parietal lobe of the cerebrum is responsible for _____.
   A. creative thinking
   B. audio signal interpretation
   C. body movement control
   D. visual signal processing

4. Which brain gland is most likely to be activated when people perceive fear?
   A. The amygdala.　　　　　　B. The hypothalamus.
   C. The thalamus.　　　　　　D. The telecephalon.

5. Memory retainment and retrieval are mainly coordinated by _____.
   A. the thalamus　　　　　　B. the frontal lobe
   C. the hippocampus　　　　　D. the basal ganglia

6. The brain delivers information to different muscles and glands through _____.
   A. afferent nerves　　　　　B. efferent nerves
   C. automatic nerves　　　　　D. visceral nerves

7. Which type of nervous system activates the fight or flight mechanism of the human body?
   A. The somatic nervous system.
   B. The parasympathetic nervous system.
   C. The sympathetic nervous system.
   D. The voluntary nervous system.

8. Association nerves perform the function of _____.
   A. conducting information to and from the brain
   B. transmitting sensory information into the spinal cord
   C. controlling the unconscious movement of visceral organs
   D. coordinating sensory input with motor output

9. The shorter outgrowths reaching out from the neuron cell body are called _____.
   A. the axon terminals　　　　B. the dendrites
   C. the sheath　　　　　　　　D. the axon

10. Why is the nervous system the most important part of the body?
    A. Because it is located in the brain.
    B. Because it is protected by the cranium and the spine.
    C. Because it controls all the other body systems.
    D. Because it controls all the biological processes and movements of the body.

II . Fill in each blank with a proper word mentioned in the text. The first letter of the word is given.

1. The simplest part of the brain that most creatures have evolved to have is the brain s_____.

2. The level of consciousness necessary for sleep is created by the p_____.

3. The body balance and equilibrium is mainly maintained by the c_____.

4. The "gray matter" of the cerebrum is called the cerebral c_____.

5. The function of interpreting audio signals received from ears is localized in the t_____ lobe of the cerebrum.

6. The information exchange between the spinal cord and the cerebrum happens in the gland of t_____.

7. The sudden, involuntary, and automatic response actions typically exhibited in case of danger are called r_____ actions.

8. As a part of the peripheral nervous system, the s_____ nervous system is involved in the control and regulation of voluntary movements.

9. Some support cells wrap around the axon to form an insulating s_____.

10. The little gap between the neurons where neurotransmitters can cross and relay signals to the neighboring cells is called the s_____.

Ⅲ. Fill in each blank in the following paragraph with a word or phrase in the box. Change the form of words if necessary.

peripheral	sensory	consciousness	unconsciousness
react	automatic	sympathetic	parasympathetic
external	visceral	brain	adapt
spinal cord	voluntary	response	

The nervous system directs the function of the body's organs and systems. It allows us to interpret what is occurring in our 1_____ environment and helps us to decide how to 2_____ to any environment change. The central nervous system (CNS) includes the brain and the 3_____. The CNS receives sensory input and produces motor responses via nerves. 4_____ nerves gather information from the environment and send that information to the spinal cord, which then sends the message to the 5_____. The brain then makes sense of that message and fires off a 6_____. Motor neurons deliver the instructions from the brain to the rest of your body. The 7_____ nervous system is divided into two categories: the somatic nervous system that controls 8_____ muscle movements and the

9_____ nervous system that functions largely below the level of 10_____ to control functions such as heart rate, respiration, and digestion.

IV. Translate the following English sentences into Chinese.

1. The nervous system consists of the central nervous system, essentially the processing area, and the peripheral nervous system which detects and sends electrical impulses in the nervous system.

2. It is the cerebrum that translates our nervous impulses into understandable quantifiable feelings and thoughts.

3. Reflex actions are those actions that are sudden, involuntary, and automatic response actions, the axon typically exhibited by humans when the survival instinct kicks in or when danger is detected.

4. On the end of the axon lie the axon terminals, which "plug" into a cell where the electrical signal from a nerve cell to the target cell can be made.

5. Due to its importance, the nervous system is safely encased within bones, namely, the cranium protecting the brain and the spine protecting the spinal cord.

V. Write a 100-word summary of the location and functions of glands in the limbic system of the cerebrum.

Reading

Text B   Diseases of the Nervous System and Their Treatment

Neurological diseases fall into the following categories: degenerative, functional, and **seizure** disorders; congenital disorders; infectious disorders; **intracranial** tumors; traumatic disorders; and cerebrovascular disorders.

Degenerative, Functional, and Seizure Disorders

Parkinson's disease is the degeneration of nerves in the brain, occurring in later life and leading to **tremors**, weakness of muscles, and slowness of movement. This slowly progressive condition is caused by a deficiency of **dopamine** that is made by cells in the midbrain. **Motor** disturbances include **stooped** posture, **shuffling gait**, muscle stiffness, and often a tremor of the hands. In patients with mild symptoms, **anticholinergic** agents and antidepressants (they block the **reuptake** of dopamine from nerve synapses) are effective. Drugs such as **levodopa** plus **carbidopa** that increase dopamine levels in the brain are useful **palliative** measures to control the most severe symptoms. In addition to drug therapy, supportive measures with physical therapy play a very important role in keeping the person's mobility maximized.

Epilepsy is a chronic brain disorder characterized by recurrent seizure activities. A seizure is an abnormal, sudden excessive **discharge** of electrical activity within the brain. Seizures are often symptoms of underlying brain pathological conditions, such as brain tumors, **meningitis**, vascular disease, or scar tissue from a head injury. **Tonic-clonic** seizures are the most common seizures in adults and children. They are characterized by a sudden loss of consciousness, falling down, and tonic contractions (stiffening of muscles) followed by clonic contractions (**twitching** and **jerking** movements of the limbs). Drug therapy (**anticonvulsants**) is used for the control of epileptic seizures.

Multiple sclerosis is a degenerative inflammatory disease of the central nervous system attacking the myelin sheath in the spinal cord and brain, leaving it **sclerosed** or scarred. Multiple sclerosis largely affects young adults aged between 20 and 40 years old, with females being affected more often than males.[1] The disease can follow two types: the **exacerbation-remitting** type in which the exacerbation or onset of symptoms is followed by a complete **remission**, or the chronic progressive type in which there is a steady loss of neurological function. **Demyelination** (scarring of the myelin sheath) prevents the conduction of nerve impulses through the axon and causes **paresthesia**, muscle weakness, unsteady gait, and **paralysis**. There may be visual and speech disturbance as well. Immunosuppressive agents are often given with some benefits.

Congenital Disorders

Hydrocephalus is an abnormal accumulation of fluid in the brain. If the circulation of cerebral spinal fluid (CSF) in the brain or spinal cord is impaired, it accumulates under pressure in the ventricles of the brain. Characteristic features in infants are an enlarged head and a small face. To relieve pressure on the brain, a **catheter** (**shunt**) is placed from the ventricle of the brain into the peritoneal space so that the CSF is continuously drained from the brain. Hydrocephalus can also occur in an adult as a result of tumors and infections.

Infectious Disorder

Meningitis is a serious bacterial infection of the **meninges** that can have **residual** debilitating effects or even a fatal outcome if not diagnosed and treated promptly with appropriate antibiotic therapy. Meningitis is caused by **meningococcal** or streptococcal bacteria or viruses. Symptoms are fever and signs of **meningeal irritation**, such as headache, **photophobia**, and a stiff neck. Antibiotics are used to treat the more serious **pyogenic** form, and the viral form is treated symptomatically until it runs its course[2]. The outcome of bacterial meningitis varies from complete recovery to[3] **miscellaneous** physical and mental disabilities. These outcomes are related to the age of the individual as well as the interval between the onset of symptoms and the beginning of treatment.

Brain Tumors

An intracranial tumor causes the normal brain tissue to be displaced and compressed, leading to progressive neurological deficiencies. The clinical symptoms of intracranial tumors include headaches, dizziness, vomiting, problems with coordination and muscle strength, and seizures.

Most of the primary intracranial tumors arise from **neuroglial** cells (**glioma**) or the meninges (**meningioma**). Examples of gliomas are **astrocytoma** and **oligodendroglioma**. The most malignant form of astrocytoma is **glioblastoma multiforme**. Meningioma and **schwannoma** are two other types of brain tumors. These tumors occur most often between 40 and 70 years of age. They are usually **noncancerous** but still may cause serious complications and death from their size or location. Surgical removal is the desired treatment for intracranial tumors. Radiation and chemotherapy are used according to location, classification, and type. Steroids are given to reduce swelling after surgery.

Traumatic Disorder

Cerebral **concussion** is a brief interruption of brain function usually with a loss of consciousness lasting for a few seconds. The **transient** loss of consciousness is usually caused by **blunt** trauma to the head. The individual experiencing a cerebral concussion is likely to have a headache after regaining consciousness and not be able to remember the events surrounding the injury. Other symptoms include blurred vision, **drowsiness**, confusion, and visual disturbances.

Cerebrovascular Disorders

A stroke occurs when the blood supply for the brain is blocked or interrupted—for example, by a blood clot, where the blood thickens and becomes solid. There are three types of strokes. Cerebral **thrombosis** makes up 50 percent of all cerebrovascular accidents and occurs largely in individuals older than 50 years of age and often during rest or sleep. The cerebral clot is typically caused by atherosclerosis, which is a thickened, **fibrotic** vessel wall that causes the vessel to be decreased in diameter or completely closed off from the buildup of plaque. Cerebral embolism occurs when an embolus or fragments of a blood clot, fat, or tumor lodge in a cerebral vessel and cause an occlusion. This occlusion renders the area supplied by this vessel **ischemic**.[4] A heart problem, such as endocarditis and atrial fibrillation, may lead to the occurrence of a cerebral embolus. Cerebral hemorrhage occurs when a cerebral vessel ruptures, allowing bleeding into the CSF, brain tissue, or the **subarachnoid** space. This type of stroke is often fatal and results from advancing age, atherosclerosis, or high blood pressure, all of which result in degeneration of cerebral blood vessels.

Symptoms of a cerebrovascular disorder may vary from going unnoticed to numbness, confusion, and dizziness, to more severe disabilities such as coma, paralysis, and **aphasia**. Three major risk factors for stroke are hypertension, diabetes, and heart disease. Thrombotic strokes are treated medically with anticoagulant drug therapy and surgically with **carotid endarterectomy**.

▶ Word Bank

seizure /ˈsiːʒə/ n.（癫痫）发作

tremor /ˈtremə/ n. 颤抖，震颤

motor /ˈməʊtə/ a. 运动神经的

shuffle /ʃʌfl/ v. 缓慢移动

anticholinergic /ˌæntɪˌkɒlɪˈnɜːdʒɪk/ a. 抗胆碱能的

levodopa /ˌliːvəˈdəʊpə/ n. 左旋多巴

palliative /ˈpælɪətɪv/ a. 减轻的，缓解的

discharge /ˈdɪstʃɑːdʒ/ n. 释放；放电；排出物

tonic-clonic /ˈtɒnɪk ˈklɒnɪk/ a. 强直阵挛性的

jerk /dʒɜːk/ v. 急动；猛拉

epileptic /ˌepɪˈleptɪk/ a. 癫痫的

sclerosis /skləˈrəʊsɪs/ n. 硬化（症）

exacerbation /ɪɡˌzæsəˈbeɪʃn/ n. 恶化，加重

remission /rɪˈmɪʃn/ n. 缓和，减轻

paresthesia /ˌpærəsˈθiːʒə/ n. 感觉异常

hydrocephalus /ˌhaɪdrəʊˈsefələs/ n. 脑积水

shunt /ʃʌnt/ n. 分流器

residual /rɪˈzɪdjʊəl/ a. 剩余的，残留的

meningeal /məˈnɪndʒɪəl/ a. 脑膜的

photophobia /ˌfəʊtəˈfəʊbɪə/ n. 畏光，恐光

miscellaneous /ˌmɪsəˈleɪnɪəs/ a. 多方面的，性质混杂的

neuroglial /njʊərəʊˈɡlɪəl/ a. 神经胶质的

intracranial /ˌɪntrəˈkreɪnɪəl/ a. 颅内的

dopamine /ˈdəʊpəmiːn/ n. 多巴胺

stoop /stuːp/ v. 弯腰，佝偻

gait /ɡeɪt/ n. 步态，步法

reuptake /riːˈʌpteɪk/ n. 再吸收，再摄取

carbidopa /ˈkɑːbɪˌdəʊpə/ n. 卡比多巴

epilepsy /ˈepɪˌlepsɪ/ n. 癫痫症

meningitis /ˌmenɪnˈdʒaɪtɪs/ n. 脑（脊）膜炎

twitch /twɪtʃ/ v. 痉挛，抽搐

anticonvulsant /ˌæntɪkənˈvʌlsənt/ n. 抗惊厥药

multiple /ˈmʌltɪpl/ a. 多发性的

sclerose /sklɪˈrəʊs/ v. 使硬化

remit /ˈriːmɪt/ v. 使缓和，减轻

demyelination /diːˌmaɪələˈneɪʃn/ n. 髓鞘脱失

paralysis /pəˈræləsɪs/ n. 瘫痪，麻痹

catheter /ˈkæθɪtə/ n. 尿液管；导管

meninges /ˈmenɪndʒɪz/ n. 脑（脊）膜

meningococcal /məˈnɪŋɡəkɒkəl/ a. 脑膜炎球菌的

irritation /ˌɪrɪˈteɪʃn/ n. 刺激；刺激物

pyogenic /ˌpaɪəʊˈdʒenɪk/ a. 生脓的，化脓的

glioma /ɡlaɪˈəʊmə/ n. 神经胶质瘤

meningioma /ˌmɪnɪndʒɪ'əʊmə/ *n.* 脑膜瘤 astrocytoma /ˌæstrəʊsaɪ'təʊmə/ *n.* 星形细胞瘤

oligodendroglioma /ˌɒlɪgəʊden'drəʊglɪəmə/ *n.* 少突神经胶质瘤

glioblastoma multiforme /ˌglɪəʊblæ'stəʊmə 'mʌltɪfɔːm/ 多形性成胶质细胞瘤

schwannoma /ʃwæ'nəʊmə/ *n.* 神经鞘瘤 noncancerous /nɒn'kænsərəs/ *a.* 非癌变的

concussion /kən'kʌʃən/ *n.* 脑震荡 transient /'trænzɪənt/ *a.* 短暂的

blunt /blʌnt/ *a.* 钝的；迟钝的 drowsiness /'draʊzɪnəs/ *n.* 昏沉，嗜睡

cerebrovascular /ˌserəbrəʊ'væskjʊlə/ *a.* 脑血管的 thrombosis /θrɒm'bəʊsɪs/ *n.* 血栓形成

fibrotic /faɪ'brɒtɪk/ *a.* 纤维化的 ischemic /ɪs'kiːmɪk/ *a.* 缺血性的

subarachnoid /ˌsʌbə'ræknɔɪd/ *a.* 蛛网膜下的 aphasia /ə'feɪzɪə/ *n.* 失语症

carotid /kə'rɒtɪd/ *n.* 颈动脉

endarterectomy /ˌendɑːtə'rektɒmɪ/ *n.*（动脉）内膜切除术

▶ Notes

1. 该句中 with females being affected more often than males 是 with + 独立主格结构，在句中作状语。独立主格结构通常由一个名词或代词加非谓语动词组成，独立主格结构中的名词或代词与其后的非谓语动词构成逻辑上的主谓关系。如果 with 后的名词或代词与分词构成主动关系，用现在分词；名词或代词与分词构成被动关系时，用过去分词。

2. It runs its course 意为病程自己结束。这个用法与 The patient heals by himself.（病人自愈。）的意思相同。course 在这里的意思为病程、疗程。如：The correlation was accentuated along with the increasing of the patients' age and the course of disease.（随着年龄增长和病程增加，两者间的相关性逐渐增加。）。又如：Treatment is supplemented with a course of antibiotics to kill the bacterium.（治疗期间辅以一个疗程的抗生素注射来杀灭细菌。）。

3. vary from…to…这个结构是医学文献中的一个常用结构，翻译时常把这个结构拆开，译为"（结构或效果）各异，包括……，甚至……"。

4. render the area supplied by this vessel ischemic 这个短语是宾补结构，其中 the area 是动词 render 的宾语，ischemic 是 the area 的补足语，用以解释说明这个区域是缺血的。supplied by this vessel 为 the area 的定语。render 这个词后经常加形容词构成宾补结构。如：render the test worthless 意为使得检查毫无价值，render the surgery exceedingly difficult 意为使得手术极其困难。

Exercises

Ⅰ. **For each of the following statements, write "T" if the statement is true and "F" if the statement is false in the blank.**

_____ 1. Neurological diseases are so complicated that they cannot be classified easily.

_____ 2. Parkinson's disease in patients with mild symptoms can be treated mainly by physical therapy.

_____ 3. The impulse conduction through the axon can be hindered by the scarring of the sheath.

_____ 4. Multiple sclerosis mainly affects young male adults.

_____ 5. Hydrocephalus can be treated by placing a catheter to drain fluid from the brain ventricles.

_____ 6. Antibiotics can effectively treat meningitis caused by bacteria or viruses.

_____ 7. Astrocytoma is a type of primary intracranial tumor.

_____ 8. A loss of consciousness can be presented both in seizures and in cerebral concussion.

_____ 9. Cerebral thrombosis occurs when cerebral vessels are occluded by fat or tumor fragments.

_____ 10. Cerebral hemorrhage accounts for the highest percentage in stroke incidence.

Ⅱ. **Match each term in Column A with its correct description in Column B. Write the corresponding letter in the blank.**

Column A	Column B
_____ 1. aphasia	A. an abnormal sensation
_____ 2. palliative	B. abnormal accumulation of fluid in the brain
_____ 3. pyogenic	C. a small abnormal patch on or inside the body
_____ 4. paresthesia	D. hardening of the myelin sheath
_____ 5. plaque	E. surgical removal of the inner lining of a clogged artery

_____ 6. endarterectomy   F. a brain disorder with recurrent seizures

_____ 7. hydrocephalus   G. inability to use language because of a brain lesion

_____ 8. astrocytoma   H. of a remedy that relieves pain without curing

_____ 9. multiple sclerosis   I. producing pus

_____ 10. epilepsy   J. a type of tumor occurring in neuroglial cells

Ⅲ. Translate the following Chinese sentences into English.

1. 除了药物治疗外，支持性治疗，如理疗也在保持病人运动能力最大化方面起着重要作用。

2. 多发性硬化是中枢神经系统的一种退行性炎症病变，累及脊髓和大脑中的髓鞘，使其硬化或形成瘢痕。

3. 细菌性脑膜炎的预后差异很大，可完全治愈，但也会出现各种各样的身体和智力残疾。

4. 脑瘤会导致正常的大脑组织移位和受挤压，引发进行性的神经缺损。

5. 脑栓塞是由于栓子或血凝块、脂肪、肿瘤的碎片滞留在脑血管内，形成血管堵塞。

Ⅳ. Think critically and then answer the following questions.

1. A 64-year-old man complains of a resting tremor that lessens with intentional movement and that causes him substantial embarrassment. What might be the appropriate diagnosis for the man, and why?

2. A 75-year-old man is brought to the doctor's office by his son with concerns over developing dementia problems. Previously, the patient had been well and was forced to retire from his job a few months ago because of worsening arthritis limiting his mobility. He has been a widower for 7 months and he lives alone. His family is worried about his safety in view of these changes. What is the likely cause of the patient's dementia?

Medicine in China

Brain-Computer Tech on March in Country

Brain-computer interface (BCI) technology is becoming more than a hypothetical phenomenon in China with some momentum gained in terms of research and development as well as applications, especially amid the country's latest call to support the cutting-edge sector.

BCI is basically a technology that enables a person to control an external device using brain signals. With vanguard applications like helping people with disabilities, the technology has been a key technological battlefield for global competition. BCI technology will be strongly supported to be an important development direction and accelerated efforts will be made to explore more application scenarios for the technology. China has already formed a well-rounded industry chain including technology and applications in BCI. Related applications have already been applied in sectors like medical care and education.

"China's BCI has been developing really fast. In some niche sectors, China stands at the same forefront with leading countries in the field," said Zhao Jizong, a renowned neurosurgical expert and academician at the Chinese Academy of Sciences. According to a report recently launched by the Brain-Computer Interface Industrial Alliance, China and the United States are important birthplaces and markets for BCI technology. China has a leading advantage in the non-implantable acquisition and sensing technology of BCI.

Applications for patents in the segment in China soared to 35 percent of the global total in recent years, followed by 30 percent from the U.S. and 10 percent from Japan, the report said.

Exercises

Ⅰ. **Translate the underlined part into Chinese.**

Ⅱ. **Answer the following question.**

In what way is China leading the world in brain-computer interface technology?

Chapter 10

Endocrine System

Pre-Reading Question

Read the following two old sayings, "Whatsoever was the father of disease, an ill diet was the mother" and "Man may be the captain of his fate, but is also the victim of his blood sugar". How do you understand the two pairs of words in them: father and mother; captain and victim?

Reading

Text A Structure and Functions of the Endocrine System

The endocrine system includes all of the glands of the body and the hormones produced by these glands. The glands are controlled directly by stimulation from the nervous system as well as by chemical receptors in the blood and hormones produced by other glands. By regulating the functions of organs in the body, these glands help to maintain the homeostasis of the body. Cellular metabolism, reproduction, sexual development, sugar and mineral homeostasis, heart rate, and digestion are among the many processes regulated by the actions of hormones.

Glands of the Endocrine System

Each gland of the endocrine system releases specific hormones into your **bloodstream**. These hormones travel through your blood to other cells and help control or coordinate many body processes. Endocrine glands (Figure 10-1) include:

- **Hypothalamus**

The hypothalamus is a part of the brain located **superior** and anterior[1] to the brain stem and **inferior** to the thalamus. It serves many different functions in the nervous system and is also responsible for the direct control of the endocrine system through the **pituitary** gland. The hypothalamus contains special cells called **neurosecretory** cells—neurons that secrete hormones such as **thyrotropin-**

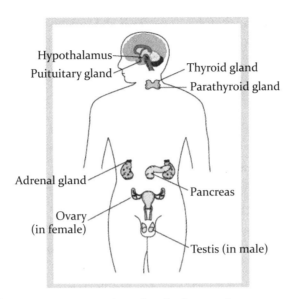

Figure 10-1   Schematic representation of major human hormone-producing organs

releasing hormone[2] (TRH), growth hormone-releasing hormone (GHRH), growth hormone-inhibiting hormone (GHIH), **gonadotropin**-releasing hormone (GnRH), **corticotropin**-releasing hormone (CRH), **oxytocin**, and **antidiuretic** hormone (ADH). All of the releasing and inhibiting hormones affect the function of the anterior pituitary gland.

- **Pituitary Gland**

The pituitary gland, also known as the **hypophysis**, is a small pea-sized **lump** of tissue connected to the inferior portion of the hypothalamus of the brain. Many blood vessels surround the pituitary gland to carry the hormones it releases throughout the body. Situated in a small **depression** in the **sphenoid** bone called the **sella turcica**, the pituitary gland is actually made of two completely separate structures: the posterior and anterior pituitary glands. The posterior pituitary gland is actually not glandular tissue at all, but nervous tissue instead. The posterior pituitary is a small extension of the hypothalamus through which the axons of some of the neurosecretory cells of the hypothalamus extend. The anterior pituitary gland is the true glandular part of the pituitary gland. The function of the anterior pituitary gland is controlled by the releasing and inhibiting hormones of the hypothalamus.

- **Pineal Gland**

The pineal gland is a small **pinecone**-shaped mass of glandular tissue found just posterior to the thalamus of the brain. The pineal gland produces the hormone **melatonin** that helps to regulate the human sleep-wake cycle known as the **circadian** rhythm. The activity of the pineal gland is inhibited by stimulation from the **photoreceptors** of the **retina**. This light sensitivity causes melatonin to be produced only in low light or darkness. Increased melatonin production causes humans to feel **drowsy** at night time when the pineal gland is active.

- **Thyroid Gland**

The thyroid gland is a butterfly-shaped gland located at the base of the neck and wrapped around the lateral sides of the trachea. The thyroid gland produces three major hormones: **calcitonin, triiodothyronine** (T3), and **thyroxine** (T4). Calcitonin is released when calcium ion levels in the blood rise above a certain set point. Calcitonin functions to reduce the concentration of calcium ions in the blood by aiding the absorption of calcium into the **matrix** of bones. The hormones T3 and T4 work together to regulate the metabolic rate of the body. Increased levels of T3 and T4 lead to increased cellular activity and energy usage in the body.

- **Parathyroid Glands**

The parathyroid glands are four small masses of glandular tissue found on the posterior side of the thyroid gland. The parathyroid glands produce the parathyroid hormone (PTH), which is involved in calcium ion homeostasis. PTH is released from the parathyroid glands when calcium ion levels in the blood drop below a set point. PTH stimulates the **osteoclasts** to break down the calcium-containing bone matrix to release free calcium ions into the bloodstream. PTH also triggers the kidneys to return calcium ions **filtered** out of the blood back to the bloodstream so that it is **conserved**.

- **Adrenal Glands**

The adrenal glands are a pair of roughly **triangular** glands found immediately superior to the kidneys. The adrenal glands are each made up of two distinct **layers**, each with its own unique functions: the outer adrenal cortex and inner adrenal medulla. The adrenal cortex produces many **cortical** hormones in three classes: glucocorticoids, **mineralocorticoids**, and **androgens**. The adrenal medulla produces the hormones **epinephrine** and **norepinephrine** under stimulation by the sympathetic division of the autonomic nervous system.

- **Pancreas**

The pancreas, a large gland located in the abdominal cavity just inferior and posterior to the stomach, is considered to be a **heterocrine** gland as it contains both endocrine and exocrine tissues. The endocrine cells of the pancreas make up just about 1% of the total mass of the pancreas and are found in small groups throughout the pancreas called **islets of Langerhans**. Within these islets are two types of cells—alpha and beta cells. The alpha cells produce the hormone **glucagon** and are responsible for raising blood glucose levels. The beta cells produce the hormone insulin, responsible for lowering blood glucose levels after a meal. Insulin triggers the absorption of glucose from the blood into cells, where it is added to glycogen molecules for storage.

- **Gonads**

The gonads—**ovaries** in females and **testes** in males—are responsible for producing the sex hormones of the body. These sex hormones determine the secondary sex characteristics of adult females and adult males. The testes, a pair of **ellipsoid** organs found in the **scrotum** of males, produce androgen **testosterone** in males after the start of **puberty**. Testosterone affects many parts of the body, including muscles, bones, sex organs, and hair **follicles**. This hormone causes growth and increases the strength of the bones and muscles, including the accelerated growth of long bones during **adolescence**. The ovaries are a pair of **almond**-shaped glands located in the pelvic cavity lateral and superior to the uterus in females. The ovaries produce the female sex hormones **progesterone** and **estrogens**.

- **Thymus**

The thymus is a soft, triangular-shaped organ found in the chest posterior to the sternum. The thymus produces hormones called **thymosins** that help to train and develop T-lymphocytes during fetal development and childhood.

In addition to the glands of the endocrine system, many other non-glandular organs and tissues in the body such as the heart, kidneys, digestive system, and **placenta** produce hormones as well.

Even the slightest **hiccup** with the function of one or more of these glands can throw off the **delicate** balance of hormones in your body and lead to an endocrine disorder, or endocrine disease.

▶ Word Bank

bloodstream /'blʌdstriːm/ n. 血流
inferior /ɪn'fɪərɪə/ a. 下部的；低劣的
neurosecretory /ˌnjʊərəʊsɪ'kriːtərɪ/ a. 神经分泌的
thyrotropin /θaɪ'rɒtrəpɪn/ n. 促甲状腺素，甲状腺刺激激素
gonadotropin /ˌɡɒnədəʊ'trɒpɪn/ n. 促性腺激素
corticotropin /ˌkɔːtɪkəʊ'trəʊpɪn/ n. 促肾上腺皮质激素，亲皮质素
oxytocin /ˌɒksɪ'təʊsɪn/ n. 后叶催产素
hypophysis /haɪ'pɒfəsɪs/ n. 脑下垂体
depression /dɪ'preʃən/ n. 下陷处

superior /sjuː'pɪərɪə/ a. 上部的，较高的
pituitary /pɪ'tjuːɪtərɪ/ n. （脑）垂体

antidiuretic /ˌæntɪdaɪjʊ'retɪk/ a. 抑制尿分泌的
lump /lʌmp/ n. 团；肿块
sphenoid /'sfiːnɔɪd/ a. 蝶骨的；楔状的

sella turcica /ˈselə ˈtɜːsɪkə/ n. 蝶鞍

pinecone /ˈpaɪnkɒn/ n. 松球，松果

circadian /sɜːˈkeɪdɪən/ a. 昼夜节奏的

photoreceptor /ˌfəʊtəʊrɪˈseptə/ n. 光感受器，感光器

drowsy /ˈdraʊzɪ/ a. 昏昏欲睡的

triiodothyronine /ˌtraɪaɪədəʊˈθaɪrənɪn/ n. 三碘甲状腺氨酸

thyroxine /θaɪˈrɒksɪn/ n. 甲状腺素，甲状腺氨酸

parathyroid /ˌpærəˈθaɪrɔɪd/ a. 副甲状腺的

filter /ˈfɪltə/ v. 过滤；滤除

conserve /kənˈsɜːv/ v. 保护，保存；使（能量）守恒

layer /ˈleɪə/ n. 层，层次

mineralocorticoid /ˌmɪnrələˈkɔːtɪkɔɪd/ n. 盐皮质激素

epinephrine /ˌepɪˈnefrɪn/ n. 肾上腺素

norepinephrine /ˌnɔːrepɪˈnefrɪn/ n. 降肾上腺素，去甲肾上腺素

heterocrine /ˈhetərəkraɪn/ a.（腺）多种分泌的

glucagon /ˈgluːkəˌgɒn/ n. 胰高血糖素，胰增血糖素

ovary /ˈəʊvərɪ/ n. 卵巢

ellipsoid /ɪˈlɪpsɔɪd/ a. 椭圆的

testosterone /teˈstɒstərəʊn/ n. 睾丸激素

follicle /ˈfɒlɪkl/ n. 小囊；卵泡；滤泡

almond /ˈɑːmənd/ n. 杏仁；扁桃

estrogen /ˈestrəʊdʒən/ n. 雌激素

thymosin /ˈθaɪməsɪn/ n. 胸腺素

hiccup /ˈhɪkʌp/ n. 打嗝；暂时性的小问题

pineal /ˈpɪnɪəl/ a. 松球状的，松果腺的

melatonin /ˌmeləˈtəʊnɪn/ n. 褪黑激素

retina /ˈretɪnə/ n. 视网膜

calcitonin /ˌkælsɪˈtəʊnɪn/ n. 降血钙素

matrix /ˈmeɪtrɪks/ n. 基质，发源地

osteoclast /ˈɒstɪəklæst/ n. 破骨细胞

triangular /traɪˈæŋɡjʊlə/ a. 三角（形）的

cortical /ˈkɔːtɪkəl/ a. 皮层的，皮质的

androgen /ˈændrɒdʒən/ n. 雄激素类

islet of Langerhans /ˈaɪlət ɒv ˈlɑːŋəˌhɑːns/ n. 胰岛

gonad /ˈɡəʊnæd/ n. 性腺

testis /ˈtestɪs/ n. 睾丸（复数为 testes）

scrotum /ˈskrəʊtəm/ n. 阴囊

puberty /ˈpjuːbətɪ/ n. 青春期

adolescence /ˌædəˈlesəns/ n. 青春期

progesterone /prəˈdʒestərəʊn/ n. 孕酮，黄体酮

thymus /ˈθaɪməs/ n. 胸腺

placenta /pləˈsentə/ n. 胎盘

delicate /ˈdelɪkət/ a. 微妙的

▶ Notes

1. superior（上部）和 anterior（前部）在医学文献中常表示解剖位置，还有 inferior（下部）、posterior（后部）、lateral（侧面）等，一般都跟介词 to 搭配。

2. thyrotropin-releasing hormone 为名词加现在分词构成复合形容词作定语，类似的还有 growth hormone-inhibiting hormone（生长激素抑制剂），thyroid-stimulating hormone test（促甲状腺激素化验）等。

Exercises

Ⅰ. **Choose the best answer to each of the following questions.**

1. What does the endocrine system include?
    A. Chemical receptors in the blood.

B. Sex organs and hormones.

C. Stimulators of the nervous system.

D. Glands and the hormones they produce.

2. What do all the glands help to maintain in the body?
   A. Metabolism.   B. Homeostasis.
   C. Reproduction.   D. Sexual development.

3. Through what does the hypothalamus directly control the endocrine system?
   A. The pituitary gland.   B. The thalamus.
   C. The neurons.   D. The hormones.

4. The pituitary gland is situated in _____.
   A. the sphenoid bone   B. the thalamus
   C. the sella turcica   D. the neck

5. Melatonin is a hormone produced by _____ to regulate the human sleep-wake cycle.
   A. the adrenal gland   B. the thyroid gland
   C. the pituitary gland   D. the pineal gland

6. What are the major hormones produced by the thyroid gland?
   A. Calcitonin, triiodothyronine, and thyroxine.
   B. Glucagon, epinephrine, and norepinephrine.
   C. Insulin, progesterone, and estrogens.
   D. Glucocorticoids, mineralocorticoids, and androgens.

7. What is the function of the parathyroid glands?
   A. To absorb calcium ions back into the blood.
   B. To help maintain calcium ion homeostasis.
   C. To release free calcium ions into the bloodstream.
   D. To conserve calcium ions in the blood.

8. The pancreas is considered to be a(n) _____.
   A. endocrine gland   B. exocrine gland
   C. heterocrine gland   D. adrenal gland

9. What do the gonads include?
   A. The ovaries and testes.
   B. The progesterones and estrogens.
   C. The scrotum and follicles.
   D. The pelvis and uterus.

10. The thymus is a soft, triangular-shaped organ found in the chest _____ to the sternum.

    A. superior   B. posterior

    C. anterior   D. inferior

Ⅱ. Match each term in Column A with its corresponding description in Column B. Write the corresponding letter in the blank.

Column A	Column B
_____ 1. hypothalamus	A. four small masses of glandular tissue
_____ 2. pituitary gland	B. a pair of roughly triangular glands
_____ 3. pineal gland	C. a small pinecone-shaped mass
_____ 4. thyroid gland	D. a large gland in the abdominal cavity
_____ 5. parathyroid glands	E. a pair of oval organs
_____ 6. adrenal glands	F. a small pea-sized lump of tissue
_____ 7. pancreas	G. a pair of almond-shaped glands
_____ 8. testes	H. a butterfly-shaped gland
_____ 9. ovaries	I. a soft, triangular-shaped organ
_____ 10. thymus	J. the lower part of the forebrain

Ⅲ. Fill in each blank in the following paragraph with a word in the box. Change the form of words if necessary.

nervous	secretion	blood	hypothalamus
endocrine	regulate	inhibit	hippocampus
receptor	production	producer	hormone
target	tissue	cell	

Hormones are produced not only by the specialized glands of internal 1_____ but also by a variety of cells throughout the body. Neurohormones, produced in the 2_____, are produced in cells throughout the 3_____ system and modulate neuronal function. Hormones that 4_____ production and maturation of cells of the hematopoietic and immune systems are made in cells of these lineages and in endothelial and mesenchymal cells. Growth-promoting and growth-5_____ hormones are produced by macrophages and mesenchymal cells. Many of these signaling molecules do not travel long distances through the 6_____ to reach target cells as classic 7_____ do but act on target cells near the producer cell or even on the 8_____ cell itself. During development, cell surface hormones may act on the cell surface 9_____ of a neighboring cell, thereby functioning as a cell-10_____communication system.

Ⅳ. **Translate the following English sentences into Chinese.**

1. The hypothalamus is a part of the brain located superior and anterior to the brain stem and inferior to the thalamus.

2. The posterior pituitary is a small extension of the hypothalamus through which the axons of some of the neurosecretory cells of the hypothalamus extend.

3. PTH also triggers the kidneys to return calcium ions filtered out of the blood back to the bloodstream so that it is conserved.

4. The pancreas, a large gland located in the abdominal cavity just inferior and posterior to the stomach, is considered to be a heterocrine gland as it contains both endocrine and exocrine tissues.

5. Even the slightest hiccup with the function of one or more of these glands can throw off the delicate balance of hormones in your body and lead to an endocrine disorder, or endocrine disease.

Ⅴ. **Write a summary (120w-150w) of the endocrine glands and hormones.**

Reading

Text B　Diseases of the Endocrine System and Their Treatment

Endocrine disorders are those that affect the endocrine system, which uses hormones to regulate the body's functions. The broad classification of the diseases is based on the hormonal secretions. They are **hypersecretion**, **hyposecretion**, and cancers or tumors of the endocrine glands.

The disorders, however, display a more complex mechanism or **pathogenesis**. There is sometimes an **interplay** of certain hormones—one hormone is hypersecreted due to the hyposecretion of another. The endocrine glands secrete a variety of hormones that regulate a variety of functions; therefore, a disorder of these glands can cause an abnormality in a number of organs. Some major endocrine disorders include thyroid problems and diabetes.

Thyroid Disorders

Through the hormones it produces, the thyroid gland influences almost all of the metabolic processes in your body. Thyroid disorders can range from a small, harmless **goiter** (enlarged gland) that needs no treatment to life-threatening cancer. The most common thyroid problems involve abnormal production of thyroid hormones. Excessive production of thyroid hormones results in' a condition known as **hyperthyroidism** while insufficient hormone production leads to **hypothyroidism**. Although the effects can be unpleasant or uncomfortable, most thyroid problems can be managed well if properly diagnosed and treated.

Hyperthyroidism is due to an overproduction of thyroid hormones, but the condition can occur in several ways: **Graves' disease** (the production of too much thyroid hormone), toxic **adenoma** (nodules that develop in the thyroid gland and begin to secrete thyroid hormones, upsetting the chemical balance in the body), and pituitary gland malfunctions or cancerous growths in the thyroid gland.

Hypothyroidism, by contrast, stems from an underproduction of thyroid hormones. Since the energy production in your body requires certain amounts of thyroid hormones, a drop in hormone production leads to lower energy levels. Causes of hypothyroidism include **Hashimoto's thyroiditis** or removal of the thyroid gland.

Hypothyroidism poses a special danger to newborns and infants. A lack of thyroid hormones in the system at an early age can lead to the development of **cretinism** (mental **retardation**) and **dwarfism** (**stunted** growth). Most infants now have their thyroid levels checked routinely soon after birth. In infants, as in adults, hypothyroidism can be due to these causes: a pituitary disorder, a defective thyroid, and a lack of the gland entirely. A hypothyroid infant is unusually inactive and quiet, has a poor appetite, and sleeps for excessively long periods of time.

Cancer of the thyroid gland is quite rare and occurs in less than 10% of thyroid nodules. You might have one or more thyroid nodules for several years before they are determined to be cancerous. People who have received radiation treatment to the head and neck earlier in life, possibly as a remedy for **acne**, tend to have a higher-than-normal risk of developing thyroid cancer.

Hashimoto's thyroiditis, also called Hashimoto's disease, is an autoimmune disease in which the immune system turns against the tissues of the body. In people with Hashimoto's, the immune system attacks the thyroid, leading to hypothyroidism. Hashimoto's symptoms may be mild at first or take years to develop. The first sign of the disease is often an enlarged thyroid, called a goiter. The goiter may cause the front of your neck to look **swollen**. A large goiter may make swallowing difficult. Other symptoms of an underactive thyroid due to Hashimoto's may include weight gain, **fatigue**, paleness or **puffiness** of the face, joint and muscle pain, constipation, inability to get warm, difficulty getting pregnant, hair loss or thinning, **brittle** hair, irregular or heavy **menstrual** periods, depression, and slowed heart rate.

There is no cure for Hashimoto's, but replacing hormones with medication can regulate hormone levels and restore your normal metabolism. The pills are available in several different strengths. The exact dose your doctor **prescribes** will depend on a number of factors, including age, weight, severity of hypothyroidism, other health problems, and other medicines that may interact with synthetic thyroid hormones. Once you start treatment, your doctor will order a lab test called a thyroid-stimulating hormone (TSH) test to monitor thyroid function and help ensure you are getting the right dose. Because thyroid hormones act very slowly in the body, it may take a few months for symptoms to go away and your goiter to shrink.

Diabetes

Symptoms of type 1 diabetes usually develop quickly, over a few days to weeks, and are caused by blood sugar levels rising above the normal range (**hyperglycemia**). You can inherit a tendency to develop type 1 diabetes, but most people with the disease have no family history of it. Type 1 diabetes requires lifelong treatment to keep blood sugar levels within a target range. There are many forms of insulin to treat diabetes. They are classified by how fast they start to work and how long their effects last. Currently, there is no way to prevent type 1 diabetes, but ongoing studies are exploring ways to prevent diabetes in those who are most likely to develop it.

Type 2 diabetes, once called non-insulin-dependent diabetes, is the most common form of diabetes. Diabetes is a number of diseases that involve problems with the hormone insulin. While[2] not everyone with type 2 diabetes is overweight, **obesity** and lack of physical activity are two of the most common causes of this form of diabetes. Combining diet, exercise, and medicine can help control your weight and blood sugar level.

Increasingly, weight loss surgery is being used as a tool to manage type 2 diabetes. That is because controlling diabetes and managing the related health risks is directly related to losing weight.[3] Diabetes treatment can include many elements like traditional medications, **alternative** medicine, and natural **remedies**. Today,

metformin is the first drug doctors usually recommend for people with type 2 diabetes who need to take medication. Inhaled insulin, insulin **pump**, and insulin **shot** are other options that can deliver medicine into your subcutaneous tissue.

▶ Word Bank

hypersecretion /ˌhaɪpəːsɪ'kriːʃən/ *n.* 分泌过多

hyposecretion /ˌhaɪpəʊsɪ'kriːʃən/ *n.* 分泌不足

pathogenesis /ˌpæθə'dʒenɪsɪs/ *n.* 发病机理

interplay /'ɪntəpleɪ/ *n.* 相互作用

goiter /'ɡɔɪtə/ *n.* 甲状腺肿

hyperthyroidism /ˌhaɪpə'θaɪrɔɪdɪzəm/ *n.* 甲状腺功能亢进

hypothyroidism /ˌhaɪpəʊ'θaɪrɔɪdɪzəm/ *n.* 甲状腺功能减退

Graves' disease /greɪvz dɪ'ziːz/ *n.* 甲状腺功能亢进，突眼性甲状腺肿

adenoma /ˌædə'nəʊmə/ *n.* 腺瘤

Hashimoto's thyroiditis /ˌhæʃɪ'məʊtəʊz ˌθaɪrɔɪ'daɪtɪs/ *n.* 淋巴瘤性（样）甲状腺肿，桥本氏甲状腺炎

cretinism /'kretɪnɪzəm/ *n.* 呆小病，愚侏病

retardation /ˌriːtɑː'deɪʃən/ *n.* 延迟，迟缓

dwarfism /'dwɔːfɪzəm/ *n.* 矮小症，矮态

stunted /'stʌntɪd/ *a.* 成长受妨碍的，矮小的

hypothyroid /ˌhaɪpəʊ'θaɪrɔɪd/ *a.* 甲状腺功能减退的

acne /'æknɪ/ *n.* 痤疮，粉刺

swollen /'swəʊlən/ *a.* 膨胀的，肿起的

fatigue /fə'tiːg/ *n.* 疲劳，疲乏

puffiness /'pʌfɪnəs/ *n.* 膨胀，肿胀

brittle /'brɪtl/ *a.* 脆的

menstrual /'menstrʊəl/ *a.* 月经的；每月的

prescribe /prɪ'skraɪb/ *v.* 开处方，给医嘱

hyperglycemia /ˌhaɪpəglaɪ'siːmɪə/ *n.* 多糖症，高血糖症

obesity /əʊ'biːsətɪ/ *n.* 肥胖（症）

alternative /ɔːl'təːnətɪv/ *a.* 两者择一的，替代的

remedy /'remədɪ/ *n.* 治疗法；补救办法

metformin /met'fɔːmɪn/ *n.* 二甲双胍

pump /pʌmp/ *n.* 泵

shot /ʃɔt/ *n.* 注射

▶ Notes

1. result in 表示因果关系，类似的词或词组还有 cause，lead to，stem from，give rise to，result from 等，灵活运用不同词组，可在写作中做到用词多样化。如：
    When we are tense, the body produces cortisol which can speed up the metabolism, resulting in stress breakouts on the skin surface and premature aging.（当我们紧张的时候，身体产生可以加快新陈代谢的皮质醇，导致皮肤表面紧张，皮肤早衰。）

2. while 在这里不是连接状语从句的从属连词，而是并列连词，意思是虽然，常用于句子开头。

3. 该句中 because controlling diabetes and managing the related health risks is 为表语从句，其中作从句主语的这两个动名词短语因被看作一个整体，所以谓语动词为第三人称单数。

Exercises

Ⅰ. **For each of the following statements, write "T" if the statement is true and "F" if the statement is false in the blank.**

　　　　　1.　The broad classification of diseases of the endocrine system is based on the secretion of hormones.

　　　　　2.　Certain hypersecreted hormones may cause the hyposecretion of other hormones.

　　　　　3.　The thyroid gland influences only the metabolic processes near the brain.

　　　　　4.　Thyroid disorders can range from an enlarged gland to life-threatening cancer.

　　　　　5.　Hyperthyroidism occurs due to an overproduction of thyroid hormones.

　　　　　6.　Patients with Hashimoto's disease often have symptoms like weight loss, fatigue, and hair loss.

　　　　　7.　Cancer of the thyroid gland is quite rare and occurs in less than 10% of thyroid nodules.

　　　　　8.　Most people with type 1 diabetes have a family history of it.

　　　　　9.　Type 2 diabetes, also called non-insulin-dependent diabetes, is the most common form of diabetes.

　　　　　10. Combining diet, exercise, and medicine can help control your weight and blood sugar level.

Ⅱ. **Complete the following sentences with a proper word mentioned in the text. The first letter of the word is given.**

1.　E_____ secretion of hormones is called hypersecretion.

2.　H_____ refers to insufficient secretion of hormones.

3.　Too much thyroid hormone results in a condition known as h_____.

4.　Hypothyroidism stems from u_____ of thyroid hormones.

5.　Lacking thyroid hormones at an early age can lead to the development of c_____.

6.　An enlarged thyroid is called a g_____, which causes the front of your neck to look swollen.

7. A lab test to monitor thyroid function and help ensure you are getting the right dose is called a thyroid-s_____ hormone test.

8. Hyperglycemia refers to the abnormally high level of blood s_____.

9. The first medication doctors usually recommend for people with type 2 diabetes is m_____.

10. Insulin pump and insulin shot are other options to deliver medicine into the s_____ tissue.

Ⅲ. **Translate the following Chinese sentences into English.**

1. 有时候激素之间相互作用，即一种激素的高分泌由另一种激素的低分泌引起。

2. 甲状腺素分泌过多导致甲状腺功能亢进，分泌不足则导致甲状腺功能减退。

3. 那些早年接受过头颈部放射治疗的患者比常人有更高的甲状腺癌变风险。

4. 桥本氏甲状腺炎不能治愈，但是利用药物进行激素替代治疗可以调节激素水平并且恢复正常新陈代谢。

5. 尽管不是每个 2 型糖尿病患者都体重超标，但肥胖和缺乏锻炼是这类糖尿病两个最常见的诱因。

Ⅳ. **Think critically and then answer the following questions.**

1. What are some of the problems that elderly people (especially females) might have as a result of decreasing hormone production?

2. Johnny, a 5-year-old boy, has a height 100% above the normal range for his age. He has been complaining of headaches and vision problems. A CT scan reveals a large pituitary tumor.
   (a) What hormone is being secreted in excess?
   (b) What condition will Johnny exhibit if corrective measures are not taken?
   (c) What is the probable cause of his headaches and visual problems?

Medicine in China

Eat Healthy Food in Moderation to Help Stay Fit

Eating simple food in moderate quantities has become a popular mantra for many Chinese people, while high-calorie intake and excessive eating have become a social problem, forcing many people to go on a diet to control their weight.

Statistics in 2022 show that more than 50 percent of Chinese people above the age of 18 are overweight. As a result, over 40 percent of Chinese people have an abnormal lipid profile and 60 percent have or need to guard against diabetes. Excess calorie intake is the main reason behind the rising levels of cholesterol, high blood pressure, and diabetes cases.

Many nutritionists say that the imbalanced nutrition pattern also plays a big role in people gaining weight. Their suggestion is to reduce the use of oil, salt, and sugar in cooking, minimize the intake of meat and eggs, and eat more vegetables, fruits, and coarse cereals.

With increasing awareness of eating healthy and with the consistent support of the government, hopefully, excessive calorie intake will soon become a thing of the past.

Exercises

Ⅰ. **Translate the underlined part into Chinese.**

Ⅱ. **Answer the following question.**

What healthy eating habits are suggested in the article?

Chapter 11

Urinary System ◀

Pre-Reading Question

Read the following quote and say what it means.

This too shall pass. Just like a kidney stone. —Hunter Madsen

Reading

Text A Structure and Functions of the Urinary System

The urinary system, also known as the **renal** system[1], performs the functions of removing **urea** and other **water-soluble** wastes from the body in the form of **urine**. The urinary system is composed of two kidneys, two **ureters**, one urinary bladder, and one **urethra** (Figure 11-1). The kidneys filter the blood to remove wastes and produce urine. The ureters, urinary bladder, and urethra together form the urinary tract, which acts as a **plumbing** system to drain urine from the kidneys, store it, and then release it during **urination**. Besides filtering and eliminating wastes from the body, the urinary system also works with the lungs, skin, and intestines to help maintain homeostasis.

The kidneys are a pair of bean-shaped organs located posterior to the parietal **peritoneum** (the membrane that lines the abdominal cavity) and touch the muscles of the back.[2] Their functions are to remove liquid waste from the blood in the form of urine; keep a stable balance of salts and other substances in the blood; and produce **erythropoietin**[3], a hormone that aids the formation of red blood cells. The kidney is composed of an outer cortex and an inner medulla. Blood enters the kidney from the outer renal cortex and filters through the inner renal medulla. Urine formation takes place in functional units called **nephrons**. The filtered urine is then **excreted** from the renal pelvis to the ureter.

There are approximately 1.25 million nephrons in each kidney. Almost 0.5 inches (1.2 centimeters) in length, each nephron begins in the lower portion of the

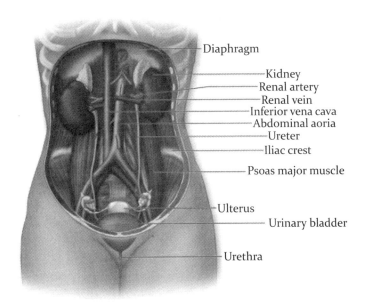

Figure 11-1   Structure of the urinary system

renal cortex, then twists and **coils** down into a renal pyramid in the renal medulla. A nephron has two major portions: a renal **corpuscle** and a renal **tubule**. The renal corpuscle is a knotted network of fine capillaries surrounded by a cup-shaped chamber. The knot of capillaries is called a **glomerulus**. The cup-shaped chamber is called the Bowman's **capsule** or **glomerular** capsule, and it is filled with fluid and has an inner wall and an outer wall. The inner wall encloses the glomerulus and has many **pores** that make it permeable or able to allow fluids or materials to pass easily through it. Its outer wall has no pores and is, thus, not permeable. The renal tubule is a long passageway that continues from the Bowman's capsule. It twists and turns down through a renal pyramid before forming a loop (called Henle's loop) and ascending back through the renal pyramid. As it ascends, it becomes slightly larger. This larger section of the renal tubule twists and coils across the top of the renal pyramid before descending once again. It then empties into a collecting duct that serves several renal tubules. Several collecting ducts then unite to form larger ducts that empty urine into a **calyx** at the tip of the renal pyramid.

Nephrons form urine in three steps: **filtration**, reabsorption, and secretion. Urine formation begins with the process of filtration, which occurs when the blood enters the glomerulus. Blood flowing through the glomeruli exerts pressure, and this glomerular blood pressure is high enough to push water, **dissolved** glucose, salt, and waste materials out of the glomeruli into the Bowman's capsule. The process by which the fluid is separated from the blood in the glomerulus is called glomerular filtration and the filtered substances are called glomerular **filtrate**. In the glomerular filtration process, large molecules, red blood cells, and platelets are unable to pass through the capillary walls. Reabsorption is the movement of substances out of the renal tubules into the blood capillaries located around the tubules. Water, glucose, and other nutrients, sodium, and other ions are substances that are reabsorbed. Reabsorption begins in the proximal **convoluted** tubules and continues in the Henle's loop, distal convoluted tubules, and collecting ducts. Secretion is the process by which substances are removed from the blood into the urine in the distal and collecting ducts. Hydrogen ions, **potassium** ions, **ammonium**, and drugs such as **penicillin** are some of the substances that are secreted from the blood into the **tubular** urine. Kidney tubule secretion plays a crucial role in maintaining the acid-base balance in the body.

The ureters are muscular tubes that carry urine from the renal pelvis to the urinary bladder. The ureters are about 10 to 12 inches long and run on the left and right sides of the body parallel to the vertebral column. Gravity and peristalsis of the smooth muscle tissue in the walls of the ureters move urine toward the urinary bladder. The ends of the ureters extend slightly into the urinary bladder and are sealed at the point of entry to the bladder by the **ureterovesical** valves. These valves prevent urine from flowing back towards the kidneys.

The urinary bladder is a hollow, **collapsible**, muscular sac that stores urine temporarily. It is located in the pelvis behind the pelvic bones and is held in place by ligaments. In women, the bladder is in front of the uterus; in men, it is above the **prostate** gland. Urine entering the urinary bladder from the ureters slowly fills the hollow space of the bladder and stretches its elastic walls. The walls of the bladder allow it to stretch to hold anywhere from 600 to[4] 800 **milliliters** of urine. The muscular walls of the urinary bladder contract to expel urine out of the bladder into the urethra. A sphincter or ring of muscle called the internal **urethral** sphincter, surrounds the opening to the urethra and controls the flow of urine. This is an involuntary sphincter, meaning a person cannot consciously control its workings.

The urethra is a thin-walled tube that carries urine from the urinary bladder to the outside of the body. Its length and function differ in females and males. In females, the urethra measures about 1 to 1.5 inches (2.5 to 3.8 centimeters) in length. Its external opening lies in front of the **vaginal** opening. The only purpose of the urethra in females is to conduct urine to the outside of the body. In males, the urethra extends from the urinary bladder through the prostate gland to the tip of the **penis**, a distance of 6 to 8 inches (15 to 20 centimeters). The urethra serves the **dual** purpose of transporting **semen** and urine to the exterior of the body, but never at the same time. Thus, it serves both the reproductive and urinary systems.

▶ Word Bank

renal /ˈriːnəl/ *a.* 肾脏的，肾的   urea /jʊˈriːə/ *n.* 尿素

water-soluble /'wɔːtə 'sɒljʊbl/ *a.* 可溶于水的

urine /'jʊərɪn/ *n.* 尿

ureter /jʊ'riːtə/ *n.* 尿管，输尿管

urethra /jʊ'riːθrə/ *n.* 尿道

plumbing /'plʌmɪŋ/ *n.* 管道系统

urination /ˌjʊərɪ'neɪʃən/ *n.* 排尿

peritoneum /ˌperɪtə'nɪəm/ *n.* 腹膜

erythropoietin /ɪˌrɪθrə'pɔɪətɪn/ *n.*（促）红细胞生成素

nephron /'nefrɒn/ *n.* 肾单位，肾元

excrete /ɪk'skriːt/ *v.* 排泄；分泌

coil /kɔɪl/ *v.* 将（绳、头发等）盘成圈

corpuscle /'kɔːpʌsəl/ *n.* 小体

tubule /'tjuːbjul/ *n.* 小管，细管

glomerulus /gləʊ'merjʊləs/ *n.* 肾小球

capsule /'kæpsjuːl/ *n.* 囊

glomerular /'glɒmerjʊlə/ *a.* 小球的；血管小球的

pore /pɔː/ *n.* 气孔；毛孔

calyx /'keɪlɪks/ *n.* 肾盏（复数为 calyxes 或 calyces）

filtration /fɪl'treɪʃən/ *n.* 过滤

dissolve /dɪ'zɒlv/ *v.* 溶解，溶化

filtrate /'fɪltreɪt/ *n.* 滤液

convolute /'kɒnvəluːt/ *v.* 旋绕

potassium /pə'tæsɪəm/ *n.* 钾

ammonium /ə'məʊnɪəm/ *n.* 铵，氨盐基

penicillin /ˌpenɪ'sɪlɪn/ *n.* 盘尼西林，青霉素

tubular /'tjuːbjʊlə/ *a.* 管状的

ureterovesical /ˌjʊəriːtəʊ'vesɪkəl/ *a.* 输尿管膀胱的

collapsible /kə'læpsəbl/ *a.* 可收缩的

prostate /'prɒsteɪt/ *n.* 前列腺

milliliter /'mɪlɪˌliːtə/ *n.* 毫升

urethral /jʊ'rɪθrəl/ *a.* 尿道的

vaginal /'vædʒɪnəl/ *a.* 阴道的

penis /'piːnɪs/ *n.* 阴茎

dual /'duːəl/ *a.* 双的；双重的

semen /'siːmən/ *n.* 精液；精子

▶ Notes

1.　also known as the renal system 在句中充当定语，修饰 the urinary system。过去分词短语 also known as 常常用于科技英语中，意思为"又称……""也被称为……""也称为……"。

2.　该句中过去分词短语 located posterior to the parietal peritoneum 作定语修饰 a pair of bean-shaped organs，意思为位于壁层腹膜后方的。posterior 为解剖学术语，意思为背后的、后部的，用于描述结构与结构之间、结构与整体之间的解剖位置关系。括号中的部分作 the parietal peritoneum 的同位语，进一步说明壁层腹膜是贴附于腹腔的一层膜。are 与 touch 为句子的谓语。

3.　erythropoietin 为促血细胞生成素，由 erythro 和 poietin 组成。构词成分 erythr/o 意思为赤、红。由 erythr/o 构成的词还有 erythrocyte（红细胞）、erythroblast（成红血细胞）、erythroleukemia（红白血病）、erythromycin（红霉素）等。-poietin 意思为促……生成素。如：leukopoietin（促白细胞生成素）。

4.　anywhere from ... to ... 意思为从……到……间的任何数量。如：Incubation lasts anywhere from 24–28 days, and seems to be temperature dependent.（孵化期为 24 到 28 天，具体取决于温度条件。）

Exercises

Ⅰ. **Choose the best answer to each of the following questions.**

1. Which of the following is a function of the urinary system?
   A. Removing waste products from the bloodstream.
   B. Storing salts and other substances from the blood.
   C. Secreting leukocytes and platelets into the blood.
   D. Regulating the digestion of glucose and proteins.

2. The two major regions of the kidney are the _____.
   A. major and minor calyces
   B. corpuscle and tubule
   C. medulla and cortex
   D. pelvis and ureter

3. The _____ is the basic functional and structural unit of the kidney.
   A. renal pyramid   B. renal medulla
   C. nephron   D. renal cortex

4. Which sequence correctly traces the path of urine after it leaves the kidneys?
   A. Ureters, urinary bladder, and urethra.
   B. Urinary bladder, ureters, and urethra.
   C. Urethra, urinary bladder, and ureters.
   D. Urinary bladder, urethra, and ureters.

5. What is the functional filtration unit in the kidney?
   A. The renal tubule.   B. The renal corpuscle.
   C. The nephron.   D. The glomerulus.

6. The fluid that enters the glomerulus is _____.
   A. the serum   B. the blood
   C. the urine   D. the tissue fluid

7. The three interrelated processes of urine formation are _____.
   A. filtration, secretion, and excretion
   B. secretion, reabsorption, and urination
   C. excretion, storage, and urination
   D. filtration, reabsorption, and secretion

8. High blood pressure in the glomeruli forces fluid to filter into _____.
   A. a renal tubule   B. the Bowman's capsule
   C. the Henle's loop   D. a collecting duct

9. Each ureter originates at the renal _____ in its respective kidney.
    A. corpuscle   B. pelvis
    C. tubule   D. pyramid

10. From the distal convoluted tubule, filtrate will then be carried to the _____.
    A. renal corpuscle   B. glomerular capsule
    C. the Henle's loop   D. collecting duct

Ⅱ. **Match each term in Column A with its corresponding description in Column B. Write the corresponding letter in the blank.**

Column A	Column B
_____ 1. glomerular filtrate	A. the liquid found in Bowman's capsule
_____ 2. cortex	B. a muscular sac located above the prostate gland in men
_____ 3. ureter	C. a basic structural and functional unit of the kidney
_____ 4. urinary bladder	D. a portion of the kidney that contains nephrons
_____ 5. urethra	E. a tube that directs urine from the urinary bladder to the outside of the body
_____ 6. sphincter	F. a small tube in a nephron
_____ 7. urea	G. a type of waste removed by the urinary system
_____ 8. nephron	H. a circular muscle that controls the flow of urine and helps keep urine from leaking
_____ 9. glomerulus	I. a ball of blood capillaries in a nephron
_____ 10. renal tubule	J. a tube that carries urine from the kidney to the urinary bladder

Ⅲ. **Fill in each blank in the following paragraph with a word in the box. Change the form of words if necessary.**

stone	urination	nephron	ureter	urea
protein	urine	kidney	secretion	bladder
urethra	blood	waste	infection	dysfunction

The urinary system is vital to maintaining good health. The urinary system is responsible for removing 1_____ and other 2_____ products from the body. It is generally recommended to drink at least eight 8-ounce glasses of water per day because water is vital to keeping the 3_____ flushed. Use the bathroom when the urge arises. Holding 4_____ for too long can weaken the 5_____ muscles and cause voiding（排尿）6_____. After 7_____, women should wipe from the front to the back to prevent a urinary tract 8_____ because the female 9_____ is an opening to the urinary tract. A healthy diet is important. A high-fat diet can result in the formation of kidney 10_____.

IV. Translate the following English sentences into Chinese.

1. Besides filtering and eliminating wastes from the body, the urinary system also works with the lungs, skin, and intestines to help maintain homeostasis.

2. The renal tubule twists and turns down through a renal pyramid before forming a loop (called Henle's loop) and ascending back through the renal pyramid.

3. The process by which the fluid is separated from the blood in the glomerulus is called the process of glomerular filtration.

4. The ureters are about 10 to 12 inches long and run on the left and right sides of the body parallel to the vertebral column.

5. The urethra serves the dual purpose of transporting semen and urine to the exterior of the body, but never at the same time.

V. Write a 100-word summary of the three processes involved in urine formation.

Reading

Text B Diseases of the Urinary System and Their Treatment

The urinary system of the body eliminates waste products that are left behind in the bowel and the blood after the body absorbs the required nutrients from the food. Any **mishap** in this system may disrupt the normal functioning of the body, resulting in several disorders and discomfort. The urinary system diseases have a wide range of severity, from minor to life-threatening. They have a wide variety of causes as well.

Urinary Tract Infections (UTIs)

Bacteria that enter the urinary tract may cause UTIs, which can affect the urethra, bladder, or even the kidneys. **Urethritis** is the inflammation of the urethra that commonly results from bacterial infection. Men and young boys are more prone to[1] develop this infection. In women, sexually transmitted diseases could also cause this condition. **Cystitis**, which is defined as the inflammation of the bladder, most commonly occurs as a result of infection but also can accompany **calculi**, tumors, or other conditions. Cystitis occurs more often in women than in men because the female urethra is shorter and closer to the anus (a source of bacteria) than in the male. **Pyelonephritis** refers to the inflammation of the renal pelvis and connective tissues of the kidneys. Pyelonephritis is usually caused by bacterial infection but also can result from viral infection, **mycosis**, calculi, tumors, pregnancy, and other conditions. Urinary tract infections are easily and effectively treated with a short course of antibiotics. However, infections can cause discomfort, with the patient experiencing painful urination (**dysuria**), a frequent urge to **urinate**, and cloudy urine.[2]

Urinary Stones

Urinary stones are small **crystallized** mineral **chunks** that may be present anywhere in the urinary tract. Depending on where a stone forms, it may be called a kidney stone, ureteral stone, or bladder stone. Kidney stones can cause pain in the back and sides, as well as blood in the urine (**hematuria**). Many kidney stones are small enough to pass **spontaneously** out of the urinary system. Larger ones (up to the size of a pearl), however, may obstruct the flow of urine and therefore, require medical attention. The condition can be treated by using **ultrasound** to **pulverize** the stones so that they can be flushed out of the urinary tract without surgery.

Glomerulonephritis

There are two categories of glomerulonephritis: acute and chronic. Acute glomerulonephritis is the most common form of kidney disease. This disorder occurs one to six weeks after a streptococcal infection and is characterized by hematuria, **oliguria**, **proteinuria**, and edema. Antibiotic therapy and bed rest are the usual treatments for acute glomerulonephritis. Recovery is often complete but it may progress to a chronic form of glomerulonephritis. Chronic glomerulonephritis is the general name for a variety of noninfectious glomerular disorders characterized by progressive kidney damage that leads to renal failure. Early stages of chronic glomerulonephritis are **asymptomatic**[3]. As the disorder progresses, hematuria, proteinuria, oliguria, and edema develop. Immune mechanisms are believed to be the major causes of chronic glomerulonephritis. Treatment aims at correcting the underlying cause of the disorder.

Urinary Incontinence

One of the most embarrassing and bothering urinary system disorders is urinary incontinence, a loss of bladder control. Some people who suffer from this disorder might get a strong urge to urinate but they cannot make it to[4] the washroom in time. Some may suffer from leaking the urine by merely coughing or sneezing. Common causes of urinary incontinence include medical conditions such as constipation or urinary tract infection. Temporary cases may be caused by drinking alcohol, drinking too much fluids, **irritated** bladder, or medications. Chronic cases could be a result of pregnancy, enlarged prostate, prostate cancer, bladder stones, or aging. The disorder can be treated with the help of bladder training, certain changes in fluid consumption and diet as a whole, physical therapy including pelvic floor exercises, and medications. For those who do not benefit from conservative treatment options, surgery could be a solution.

Chronic Renal Failure (CRF)

Chronic renal failure is a slow, progressive decline in the normal functioning of the kidney. The organ gradually loses its ability to remove wastes, concentrate urine, and conserve electrolytes. There are dozens of diseases that may result in the gradual loss of nephron function, including diabetes, hypertension, enlarged prostate, cancer of the bladder, cancer of the kidneys, stones in the kidneys, and lupus, to name a few[5]. Fatigue, swelling, hiccups, high blood pressure, **nausea**, headache, loss of appetite, **itching**, bad breath, nail problems, seizures, confusion, and drowsiness are the most common symptoms. The condition has no cure, but treatments help in reducing the severity of the symptoms and delaying its progress. The treatment concentrates on dealing with the underlying cause of the disease and addressing its complications.

End-stage Renal Disease (ESRD)

When the kidneys almost or completely cease to function, the condition is known as an ESRD. The symptoms are similar to those of chronic renal failure. Procedures such as **dialysis** and organ **transplant** are required for the treatment as at this stage the kidneys lose about 85% of their functioning.

Tumors

Tumors of the urinary system typically obstruct urine flow, possibly causing **hydronephrosis** in one or both kidneys. Most kidney tumors are malignant neoplasms called renal cell **carcinoma** (RCC). They usually occur only in one kidney. RCC metastasizes most often to the lungs and bone tissue. Bladder cancer occurs as frequently as renal cancer (each accounts for about two out of every hundred cancer cases) and is often found in association with bladder stones. Renal and bladder cancers have few symptoms early in their development, other than hematuria. As the cancer develops, pelvic pain and symptoms of urinary obstruction may occur. **Insertion** of a **cystoscope** through the urethra and into the bladder permits direct inspection, biopsy, and surgical removal or treatment of the bladder and other urinary tract lesions.

▶ **Word Bank**

mishap /'mɪshæp/ *n.* 小灾难

cystitis /sɪ'staɪtɪs/ *n.* 膀胱炎

pyelonephritis /ˌpaɪələʊnɪ'fraɪtɪs/ *n.* 肾盂肾炎

dysuria /dɪs'jʊrɪə/ *n.* 排尿困难

crystalized /'krɪstəlaɪzd/ *a.* 结晶的

hematuria /ˌhiːmə'tjuːrɪə/ *n.* 血尿症；血尿

ultrasound /'ʌltrəsaʊnd/ *n.* 超声；超音波

oliguria /ˌɒlɪ'gjʊərɪə/ *n.* 少尿

asymptomatic /ˌeɪsɪmptə'mætɪk/ *a.* 无症状的

irritated /'ɪrɪteɪtɪd/ *a.* 发炎的

itching /'ɪtʃɪŋ/ *n.* 痒

transplant /'trænsplɑːnt/ *n.* 移植；移植器官

carcinoma /ˌkɑːsɪ'nəʊmə/ *n.* 癌

cystoscope /'sɪstəskəʊp/ *n.* 膀胱镜

urethritis /ˌjʊərə'θraɪtɪs/ *n.* 尿道炎

calculus /'kælkjʊləs/ *n.* 结石（复数为 calculi）

mycosis /maɪ'kəʊsɪs/ *n.* 霉菌病

urinate /'jʊrɪneɪt/ *v.* 排尿

chunk /tʃʌŋk/ *n.* 大块

spontaneously /spɒn'teɪnɪəslɪ/ *ad.* 自发地，自然地

pulverize /'pʌlvəraɪz/ *v.* 粉碎，使成粉末

proteinuria /ˌprəʊtiː'njʊərɪə/ *n.* 蛋白尿

incontinence /ɪn'kɒntɪnəns/ *n.* 失禁

nausea /'nɔːzɪə/ *n.* 恶心，作呕

dialysis /ˌdaɪ'æləsɪs/ *n.* 透析；渗析

hydronephrosis /ˌhaɪdrənɪ'frəʊsɪs/ *n.* 肾盂积水

insertion /ɪn'sɜːʃən/ *n.* 插入

▶ Notes

1.　形容词短语 be prone to 意思为易于受某事物影响或做某事的。该短语中 to 是介词，后面跟名词、动词原形或者动名词。如：He was prone to anger.。

2.　with/without + 名词 / 物主代词 + 现在 / 过去分词结构为独立主格结构，在句中作伴随状语。本句中 the patient 为现在分词 experiencing 的逻辑主语。如：I stood in front of her, with my heart beating fast.。

3.　asymptomatic 前缀为 a-。a- 和 an-（用于元音音素前）可表示"无"的意思，比如：asymptomatic 无症状的、abacteria 无菌的、anemia 贫血；表示"非"的否定意思，比如：asymmetrical 不对称的、asystole 心搏停止（心脏不收缩）；表示"离开"的意思，比如：aberrant 迷走的（即离开正常途径的）。元音前用 an-，如：anesthesia 无感觉，麻醉、analgesia 无痛法，痛觉消失。

4. 短语动词 make it to 意思为到达，及时赶到。其中 to 为介词，后面跟名词或动名词。如：Some products, like some soft drinks, make it to every village in the world.

5. to name a few 一般用于句末，意思为等等，仅举几例。例如：Your nutrition choices affect your metabolism, sleep, mental acuity, stamina, and happiness, just to name a few.（你选择摄入的营养将影响到你的新陈代谢、睡眠、精神敏度、耐力和幸福感等情况。）

Exercises

Ⅰ. **For each of the following statements, write "T" if the statement is true and "F" if the statement is false in the blank.**

_____ 1. Both men and women can suffer from urethritis.

_____ 2. Immediate surgery is needed to remove the stones from the urinary tract.

_____ 3. Biopsy can examine and remove suspected tissues or liquids in the urinary system.

_____ 4. Pyelonephritis is an inflammation that usually involves multiple nephrons.

_____ 5. Chronic renal failure is reversible if the primary problem is treated successfully.

_____ 6. Acute glomerulonephritis can be cured.

_____ 7. Chronic glomerulonephritis occurs six weeks after a streptococcal infection.

_____ 8. Urinary incontinence is typically found among children and elderly people.

_____ 9. People have no symptoms at the early stage of chronic glomerulonephritis.

_____ 10. People with end-stage renal disease lose almost all their renal function.

Ⅱ. **Fill in each blank with a proper word mentioned in the text. The first letter of the word is given.**

1. Urinary tract infections are self-limiting and easily treated with a_____.

2. Urinary i_____ can range from an occasional leakage of urine to a complete inability to hold any urine.

3. Kidney stones may block the flow of u_____ and can be broken up by using ultrasound.

4. H_____ is the presence of red blood cells in the urine.

5. O_____ is the excretion of an abnormally small volume of urine.

6. P_____ is the presence of excessive protein in the urine.

7. Painful or difficult u_____ is termed as dysuria.

8. Women tend to get c_____ more often because their urethra is shorter and closer to the anus.

9. D_____ or organ transplant is required for the treatment of end-stage renal disease.

10. The most common type of kidney cancer is renal cell c_____.

Ⅲ. **Translate the following Chinese sentences into English.**

1. 食物中所需的营养物质被人体吸收后，残留在肠和血液中的废物由人体的泌尿系统排出。

2. 然而感染会导致患者尿痛（排尿困难）、尿频、尿急等不适，以及尿混浊。

3. 根据其形成位置，尿结石可被称为肾结石、输尿管结石或膀胱结石。

4. 该病可以通过膀胱训练、液体饮用及饮食习惯的改变、骨盆底锻炼等物理疗法及药物进行治疗。

5. 通过尿道将膀胱镜插入膀胱可以直接进行望诊、活组织检查和手术切除或治疗膀胱及其他泌尿道病变。

Ⅳ. **Think critically and then answer the following questions.**

1. Li Juan volunteered to teach at a primary school in a mountainous area. A few days after her arrival, she began to feel pain when she urinated. She also noticed that she went to the toilet more frequently and that her urine smelt funny and was cloudy. What might her problem be?

2. After having run 5000 meters on a very hot day, Wang Hong went to the bathroom to urinate and noticed that there was a very small amount of urine and the color was deep amber（琥珀色的）. What happened to him?

Medicine in China

Chinese Medical Equipment Transforms Treatment in South Sudan's Main Hospital

Joel Lukau Barnaba, a 73-year-old director of radiology at Juba Teaching Hospital in South Sudan, would have long been retired but due to the shortage of radiologists, he is able to diagnose about 50 patients on a daily basis with the help of Chinese medical equipment.

Lukau, who has 43 years of medical experience, told Xinhua that the creatinine clearance test (CR), computed tomography (CT) scan, and fluoroscopy donated by the Chinese government in 2019 have transformed the radiology department.

"With the help of China, now we are able to do so many things," he said while in the radiology department housed in the outpatient ward built by the Chinese government.

Lukau said he is grateful to work alongside Zhou Fengchun, a 55-year-old senior medical consultant from the ninth batch of the Chinese medical team who does differential diagnoses on patients. In addition, Zhou does remote consultation sharing scanned images of patients with colleagues at the Second People's Hospital in Anhui Province who help with proper examination and diagnosis. Zhou also jointly works with his South Sudanese colleagues to conduct CT scans on patients who turn up with kidney, liver, and bladder problems.

"Zhou is a senior consultant. When he sits with our radiologists here, he provides them with more knowledge, they should be much attached to him," says Lukau.

Exercises

Ⅰ. **Translate the underlined part into Chinese.**

Ⅱ. **Answer the following question.**

How did the Chinese medical team help the local hospital in South Sudan?

Chapter 12

Lymphatic and Immune System

Pre-Reading Question

Read the following quote and say what it means.

"There is nothing more galling to angry people than the coolness of those people on which they wish to vent their spleen." —*Alexander Dumas*

Reading

Text A   Structure and Functions of the Lymphatic and Immune System

The lymphatic system and immunity are intricately linked in that the lymphatic system is an important part of the immune system. The immune system is a group of organs and associated structures that help protect the body from possible **intruders**. These intruders come in the form of foreign bodies, most typically referred to as **antigens**. Immune cells and antibodies circulate in the bloodstream and lymphatic vessels, seeking out the pathogens to destroy them.

To best understand the relationship between the lymphatic system and immunity, it is important to develop an understanding of each system individually. As shown in Figure 12-1, the major components of the lymphatic system include the lymph, lymphatic capillaries and vessels, lymphatic nodes, and lymphatic organs (such as the thymus, red bone marrow, spleen, and **tonsils**) that contain **lymphoid** tissues. The lymphatic system maintains fluid balance in tissues, absorbs fats from the small intestine, and defends against microorganisms and foreign substances.

The cardiovascular system plays a key role in bringing many needed substances to cells and then removing the waste products that accumulate as a result of metabolism. This exchange of substances between the blood and tissue fluid occurs in capillary beds. Many additional substances that cannot enter or return through the capillary walls, including excess fluid and protein molecules, are returned to the blood as lymph. Lymph is formed when the **interstitial** fluid (the fluid which lies in the **interstices** of all body tissues) is collected through lymph capillaries. Afferent lymphatic vessels carry lymph away from tissues to lymphatic nodes. Valves in the vessels ensure the one-way flow of the lymph. After the lymph is filtered, it leaves the lymph node via an efferent lymphatic vessel, traveling toward even larger vessels called lymphatic trunks that are formed by the **confluence** of lymphatic vessels. The lymph empties ultimately into the right or the left **subclavian** vein, where it mixes back with the blood. Lymphatic vessels are found in most of the organs and tissues of the body, but they are not found in the eyeball, epidermis, cartilage, or bone marrow. The central nervous system has no lymphatic vessels, either—extra fluid drains into the cerebral spinal fluid.

Lymphoid tissue produces lymphocytes, when exposed to foreign substances, and it filters lymph and blood. In addition to being present in the lymph nodes, lymphatic tissue is also found in other lymphoid organs, such as the thymus, spleen, and tonsils. Lymphoid organs are important structural components of the immune system because they provide immune defense and the development of immune cells. The lymph nodes, located along the lymphatic vessels, function as filters of the lymph that enters from several afferent lymphatic vessels. Tonsils, located in the upper throat region, house lymphocytes and other white blood cells called macrophages. These immune cells protect the digestive tract and lungs from disease-causing agents that enter the mouth or nose. The spleen is the largest lymphoid organ in the body, located in the upper left quadrant of the abdomen lateral to the stomach. The red **pulp** of the spleen **phagocytizes** foreign substances and worn-out **erythrocytes**. The white pulp coexists and **interweaves** with red pulp and is most frequently found surrounding the arterioles of the spleen. The white pulp is made of lymphatic tissue and contains many T lymphocytes (T cells), B lymphocytes (B cells), and macrophages for fighting off infections. The spleen also functions as a **reservoir** for blood. The thymus is located just posterior to the sternum and anterior to the heart. Its primary function is to promote the **maturation** and **differentiation** of T lymphocytes, which move to other lymphatic tissues to respond to foreign substances.

Many organs in the lymphatic system provide defense: lymph nodes, tonsils, thymus, and spleen (Figure 12-1). The immune system is not simply a small group of organs working together. Instead, it is an interactive network of many organs and billions of freely moving cells, and trillions of free-floating molecules in many different areas of the body. The immune system is made up of leukocytes (white blood cells), proteins, tissues, and organs, including those of the lymphatic system. The immune system works to protect us from disease-causing microorganisms that invade our bodies, from foreign tissue cells that may have been transplanted into our bodies, and from our own cells when they have turned malignant or cancerous.

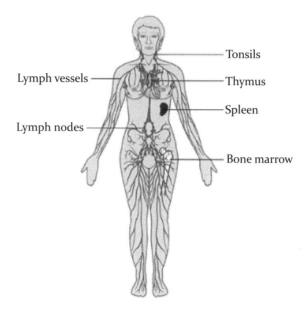

Figure 12-1   Principal organs of the lymphatic system

All leukocytes are produced and derived from **multipotent** cells in the bone marrow known as **hematopoietic** stem cells. Leukocytes are found throughout the body, including the blood and lymphatic system. Leukocytes can be further broken down into two groups based on the types of **primitive** stem cells that produce them: **myeloid** stem cells and lymphoid stem cells. Myeloid stem cells produce **monocytes** and **granular** leukocytes. Monocytes are **agranular** leukocytes, from which macrophages and **dendritic** cells are derived. Monocytes respond slowly to infection, and once present at the site of infection, develop into macrophages.[1] Macrophages are phagocytes which are able to consume pathogens, destroyed cells, and debris by **phagocytosis**. As such[2], they have a role in both preventing infection and cleaning up the **aftermath** of an infection. Monocytes also develop into dendritic cells in healthy tissues of the skin and mucous membranes. Dendritic cells are responsible for the detection of pathogenic antigens which are used to activate T cells and B cells.

There are three types of **granulocytes**: **eosinophils**, **basophils**, and **neutrophils**. As seen under a microscope, **granules** in these white blood cells are apparent when **stained**. Eosinophils are granular leukocytes that reduce allergic inflammation and help the body fight off parasites. Basophils trigger inflammation by releasing the chemicals **heparin** and **histamine**. Basophils are active in producing inflammation during allergic reactions and parasitic infections. Neutrophils act as the first responders to the site of an infection, use **chemotaxis** to detect chemicals produced by infectious agents, and quickly move to the site of the infection. Once there, neutrophils **ingest** the pathogens via phagocytosis and release chemicals to trap and kill the pathogens.

Lymphoid stem cells produce T cells and B cells. T cells and B cells start the war against antigens and foreign invaders such as bacteria or viruses in the body. When antigens are detected by any of the lymphocytes, B cells are stimulated to produce antibodies, which are proteins that attach themselves to those antigens. Together they form complexes called antigen-antibody complexes. Although the antibodies find the antigens, they cannot kill them; instead, they neutralize the pathogens until T cells call in phagocytes to help finish off the invaders. The antibodies stay in your body, so if the antigens are specifically targeted for return, they are ready to destroy these antigens as soon as they show up.

▶ Word Bank

intruder /ɪn'truːdə/ *n.* 入侵者，闯入者

antigen /'æntɪdʒən/ *n.* 抗原

tonsil /'tɒnsɪl/ *n.* 扁桃体

lymphoid /'lɪmfɔɪd/ *a.* 淋巴的；淋巴样的

interstitial /ˌɪntə'stɪʃəl/ *a.* 间质的；空隙的

interstice /ɪn'tɜːstɪs/ *n.* 间隙，缝

confluence /'kɒnfluəns/ *n.* 汇合

subclavian /sʌb'kleɪvɪən/ *a.* 锁骨下的

pulp /pʌlp/ *n.* 髓的；果肉

phagocytize /ˌfæɡəʊ'saɪtaɪz/ *v.* 吞噬

erythrocyte /ɪ'rɪθrəʊsaɪt/ *n.* 红血球，红细胞

interweave /ˌɪntə'wiːv/ *v.* 交织；混杂

reservoir /'rezəvwɑː/ *n.* 水库；蓄水池

maturation /ˌmætjʊ'reɪʃən/ *n.* 成熟

differentiation /ˌdɪfəˌrenʃɪ'eɪʃən/ *n.* 变异，分化

multipotent /ˌmʌltɪ'pəʊtənt/ *a.* 有多种能力的

hematopoietic /ˌheməˌtəʊpɔɪ'iːtɪk/ *a.* 造血的，生血的

primitive /'prɪmɪtɪv/ *a.* 原始的

myeloid /'maɪəlɔɪd/ *a.* 骨髓的；骨髓状的

monocyte /'mɒnəʊsaɪt/ *n.* 单核细胞

granular /'ɡrænjʊlə/ *a.* 颗粒的；粒状的

agranular /ə'ɡrænjʊlə/ *a.* 无颗粒的

dendritic /den'drɪtɪk/ *a.* 树枝状的

phagocytosis /ˌfæɡəʊsaɪ'təʊsɪs/ *n.* 吞噬作用

aftermath /'ɑːftəmæθ/ *n.* 后果，余波

granulocyte /'ɡrænjʊˌləsaɪt/ *n.* 粒细胞

eosinophil /ˌiːəʊ'zɪnəfɪl/ *n.* 嗜酸性细胞；嗜酸粒细胞

basophil /'beɪsəʊfɪl/ *n.* 嗜碱粒细胞

neutrophil /'njuːtrəfɪl/ *n.* 中性粒（白）细胞

granule /'ɡrænjuːl/ *n.* 颗粒

stain /'steɪn/ *v.* 染色

heparin /'hepərɪn/ *n.* 肝素

histamine /'hɪstəmiːn/ *n.* 组胺

chemotaxis /ˌkiːmə'tæksɪs/ *n.* 趋药性

ingest /ɪn'dʒest/ *v.* 咽下；吸收

▶ Notes

1. 该句主语为 monocytes, 谓语有两个，分别是 respond slowly to 和 develop into。once present at the site of infection 在句中作时间状语，状语中省略了代词 they （状语从句中的主语）和系动词 are，这是因为当并列句中两个分句主语相同时可省去第二个分句中的主语，将其补充完整就是 once they are present at the

site of infection, monocytes develop into macrophages.。

2. As such 意思为正因为如此。如：As such, I had to give up the conventional treatment and turn to target therapy.（正因如此，我不得不放弃常规治疗而进行靶向治疗。）

Exercises

Ⅰ. **Choose the best answer to each of the following questions.**

1. A major function of the lymphatic system is to _____.
   A. transport nutrients and oxygen to body tissues
   B. regulate temperature, fluid, electrolytes, and pH balance
   C. remove carbon dioxide and waste products from tissues
   D. produce, maintain, and distribute lymphocytes

2. What is the largest lymphoid organ?
   A. The thymus gland. 　　　　　B. The tonsil.
   C. The adult spleen. 　　　　　D. The lymphatic node.

3. What is located in the throat and defends against invading bacteria coming in through the mouth and nose?
   A. The thymus. 　　　　　B. The lymph.
   C. The tongue. 　　　　　D. The tonsil.

4. Lymphatic vessels transport _____ to the general circulation.
   A. tissue fluid 　　　　　B. proteins
   C. fats 　　　　　D. nutrients

5. Lymph fluid is returned into general circulation by draining into the _____.
   A. subclavian arteries
   B. subclavian veins
   C. internal thoracic arteries
   D. internal thoracic veins

6. To assist the lymph in returning to the cardiovascular system, lymph vessels _____.
   A. possess mini-pumps that drive lymph forward
   B. possess valves, like veins, to prevent backflow
   C. rely on the pressure generated by their muscular walls
   D. rely on the blood pressure generated by the heart

7.   Where do all the cells of the immune system arise from?
     A. Cells in the lymphoid nodes.
     B. Primitive cells in the thymus.
     C. Primitive cells in the bone marrow.
     D. Cells located primarily in the brain.

8.   Neutrophils and lymphocytes are types of _____.
     A. platelets   B. plasma cells
     C. white blood cells   D. red blood cells

9.   Precursors of macrophages are called _____.
     A. T cells   B. B cells
     C. plasma cells   D. monocytes

10. Which type of cells produce antibodies?
     A. B lymphocytes.   B. T lymphocytes.
     C. Monocytes.   D. Phagocytes.

Ⅱ. **Fill in each blank in the following paragraph with a word in the box. Change the form of words if necessary.**

cardiovascular	lymph	metabolism	thymus
separately	lymphatic	blood	artery
vein	lymphocyte	valve	spleen
circulation	together	tissue	

Our body actually has two circulatory systems: the lymphatic and cardiovascular systems. The 1_____ system provides our body 2_____ with the needed oxygen, nutrients, and hormone-rich blood required for everyday functions. The 3_____ system rids our body of the waste products (including old red blood cells) produced as the result of 4_____, thus protecting us from the harmful effects we would experience otherwise. While they perform their main functions, they also work 5_____ to some degree. Portions of the blood help create the 6_____, which removes wasteful 7_____ cells from the body. In addition, the 8_____ also serves as a blood reservoir for the cardiovascular system until the blood is needed. Just like the cardiovascular 9_____, the lymph vessels have one-way 10_____ to prevent backflow of the lymph.

Ⅲ. **Translate the following English sentences into Chinese.**

1.　The lymphatic system and immunity are intricately linked in that the lymphatic system is an important part of the immune system.

2.　The spleen is the largest lymphoid organ in the body, located in the upper left quadrant of the abdomen lateral to the stomach.

3.　The immune system works to protect us from disease-causing microorganisms that invade our body, from foreign tissue cells that may have been transplanted into our bodies, and from our own cells when they have turned malignant or cancerous.

4.　Monocytes are agranular leukocytes, from which macrophages and dendritic cells are derived.

5.　Neutrophils act as the first responders to the site of an infection, use chemotaxis to detect chemicals produced by infectious agents, and quickly move to the site of the infection.

Ⅳ. **Write a 100-word summary of the functions of the lymphatic system.**

Reading

Text B　Diseases of the Lymphatic and Immune System and Their Treatment

Most health problems can be linked to a poor or weak lymphatic and immune system. The lymphatic and immune system consists of organs and body tissues that produce, store, and carry disease-fighting white blood cells. In a healthy immune system, a war is being successfully **waged** against antigens and foreign substances attacking the body. However, when an immune system is losing the battle, a person can suffer various diseases and disorders.

Acquired Immune Deficiency Syndrome (AIDS)

AIDS is caused by the human **immunodeficiency** virus or HIV. Once infected, individuals may not show signs of the disease for as many as ten years or more. HIV impairs the body's ability to produce an immune response. Specifically, the virus infects helper T cells. Once inside a helper T cell, HIV can **replicate** or reproduce within the cell and kill it in ways that are still not completely understood. When the newly formed viruses break out of the dying helper T cell, they continue the cycle by infecting other helper T cells. In response, the body produces more helper T cells, but this only provides the viruses with more hosts in which to grow and spread.[1]

Because helper T cells play a central role in directing the immune response of the body, their destruction brings about a drop in cell-mediated[2] immunity. The number of antibodies produced in the body declines, leaving it without defenses against a wide range of invaders. Many different types of infections and cancers can develop, taking advantage of the weakened immune response of the body. Because their immune systems are deficient, AIDS patients usually die from one of these infections or cancers.

HIV is transmitted between humans via blood, semen, and vaginal secretions. There is currently no cure for the disease and no vaccine to prevent its spread. The best defense against AIDS is avoiding sexual contact with infected individuals. Intravenous drug use (injecting drugs into the bloodstream) of any kind should always be avoided. Several **antiviral** drugs have been developed to slow the progress of the disease in infected individuals. Combinations of these drugs—known informally as **cocktails**—have proven effective in improving the quality and length of life of AIDS patients, especially those who have been diagnosed in the early stages of the disease.

Severe Combined Immunodeficiency (SCID)

SCID represents a group of rare, sometimes fatal, congenital disorders characterized by little or no immune response. The defining feature of SCID is a defect in the specialized white blood cells (B and T lymphocytes) that defend us from infection by viruses, bacteria, and fungi. Without a functional immune system, SCID patients are susceptible to recurrent[3] infections such as pneumonia, meningitis, and **chicken pox**, and can die before the first year of life. New treatments such as bone marrow and stem cell transplantation save as many as 80% of SCID patients. Advances in using gene therapy have also been made in treating SCID patients.

Autoimmune Diseases

Autoimmune diseases are those in which the body produces antibodies and T cells that attack and damage the normal cells of the body, causing tissue destruction. Graves' disease, also called hyperthyroidism, occurs when an antibody binds to specific cells in the thyroid gland, forcing them to secrete excess thyroid hormone. Symptoms of the condition include weight loss with increased appetite, shortness of breath, tiredness, weak muscles, anxiety, and visible enlargement of the thyroid gland. Treatments include drugs to stop hormone production, **radioactive iodine** to destroy the hormone-producing cells and shrink the enlarged gland, and surgery to remove a part or all of the thyroid.[4]

Systemic lupus erythematosus (also called lupus or SLE) is a disease in which antibodies begin to attack the tissues and organs of the body as if they were foreign. The cause of SLE is unknown. It can affect both men and women of all ages, but 90 percent of those afflicted are women. Among the many symptoms of the disease are fever, weakness, muscle pain, weight loss, skin **rashes**, joint pain, headaches, vomiting, diarrhea, and inflammation of the lining of the lungs or the lining around the heart. Pink rashes on the face and arms are typically seen in cases of SLE. Treatment for SLE depends on how severe the symptoms are. Mild symptoms like inflammation can be treated with **aspirin** or **ibuprofen**. Severe symptoms are often treated with stronger drugs, including steroids. Drugs to decrease the body's immune response may also be used for severely ill SLE patients.

Lymphoma

Lymphomas, which make up about 3 percent of all cancers, refer to cancers that begin in the lymphatic system. Just like all cancers, lymphomas are diseases in which cells grow at abnormally rapid rates. The cause of lymphoma is uncertain, but it is believed to be caused by drugs taken to **suppress** the immune system. Lymphomas are divided into Hodgkin's disease (HD), also known as Hodgkin's lymphoma, and non-Hodgkin's lymphomas.

Hodgkin's lymphoma can occur at any age, although people in early adulthood (ages 15 to 34) and late adulthood (after age 60) are most affected. The cancer begins in a lymph node (usually in the neck), causing swelling and possibly pain. After affecting one group of nodes, it progresses on to the next. In advanced cases of cancer, the spleen, liver, and bone marrow may also be affected. Symptoms include fatigue, weight loss, night sweats, and itching. As the cancer spreads throughout the body, the immune response becomes less effective. Common infections caused by bacteria and viruses begin to take over. Once detected in the body, Hodgkin's disease is usually treated with chemotherapy, radiotherapy, or a combination of both.

Non-Hodgkin's lymphomas encompass over 29 types of lymphomas. Again, the exact causes of these lymphomas are unknown. Symptoms of non-Hodgkin's lymphomas are similar to those of Hodgkin's lymphoma. Apart from the swelling of lymph nodes, patients may experience loss of appetite, weight loss, nausea, vomiting, pain in the lower back, headaches, fever, and night sweats. The liver and spleen may enlarge as well. Immune responses may be weakened. Treatments for non-Hodgkin's lymphomas also include chemotherapy and radiation therapy (either by themselves or in combination). In severe cases, bone marrow transplants may be required. Since the cure rate for non-Hodgkin's lymphomas is not as good as it is for Hodgkin's lymphoma, early detection and treatment are vital.

▶ Word Bank

wage /weɪdʒ/ *v.* 进行；发动

replicate /'replɪkeɪt/ *v.* 复制

cocktail /'kɔkteɪl/ *n.* （尤指不太容易融合的几种物品的）混合物

chicken pox /'tʃɪkɪn pɒks/ *n.* 水痘

iodine /'aɪədaɪn/ *n.* 碘

aspirin /'æspərɪn/ *n.* 阿司匹林

suppress /sə'pres/ *v.* 抑制

immunodeficiency /ɪˌmju:nəʊdɪ'fɪʃənsɪ/ *n.* 免疫缺陷

antiviral /ˌæntɪ'vaɪrəl/ *a.* 抗病毒的

radioactive /ˌreɪdɪəʊ'æktɪv/ *a.* 放射性的，有辐射的

rash /ræʃ/ *n.* 皮疹

ibuprofen /ˌaɪbju:'prəʊfen/ *n.* 异丁苯丙酸；布洛芬

▶ Notes

1. in which to grow and spread 为介词 + which/whom + 不定式结构，在句中作 more hosts 的定语，more hosts 作介词 in 的宾语。本结构可扩展为定语从句 this only provides the viruses with more hosts in which the viruses grow and spread。此结构中的介词只能放在 which/whom 的前面，不可以放在不定式中的动词后。

2. 医学英语中 -mediated 常常和其他词一起构成复合形容词作定语，意思为"……介导的"。cell-mediated immunity 意思是细胞介导的免疫。又如：T-cell mediated reaction（T 细胞介导反应），antibody-mediated rejection（抗体介导性排斥反应）。

3. 形容词短语 susceptible to 意思为易受……影响的，易受（伤）的，易患（病）的，其中 to 是介词，后面跟名词或动名词。如：But what we don't know is why they become susceptible to this host of pathogens, viruses, and fungus.（但是我们不知道的是为什么他们会对这些病原菌、病毒和真菌这么敏感。）

4. 该句中三个不定式短语 to stop the hormone production, to destroy the hormone-producing cells and shrink the enlarged gland 以及 to remove a part or all of the thyroid 作后置定语分别修饰名词 drugs、radioactive iodine 及 surgery。

Exercises

Ⅰ. **For each of the following statements, write "T" if the statement is true and "F" if the statement is false in the blank.**

_____ 1. Acquired immune deficiency syndrome causes inadequate T cell formation.

_____ 2. A person infected with HIV may not show signs of AIDS.

_____ 3. Cocktails are alcoholic drinks specially mixed for the effective treatment of AIDS.

_____ 4. Most patients with severe combined immunodeficiency can be cured by bone marrow or stem cell transplantation.

_____ 5. One will get AIDS by sharing foods or drinks with an HIV-infected person.

_____ 6. Graves' disease is characterized by excess secretion of thyroid hormone.

_____ 7. Autoimmune diseases are caused by a defect in B and T lymphocytes.

_____ 8. Lupus, also known as SLE, is a congenital disease of unknown cause.

_____ 9. Hodgkin's disease may be related to drugs taken to suppress the immune system.

_____ 10. Patients with non-Hodgkin's lymphomas may have weakened immune responses.

Ⅱ . **Match each term in Column A with its correct description in Column B. Write the corresponding letter in the blank.**

Column A	Column B
_____ 1. syndrome	A. the virus that causes AIDS
_____ 2. immunodeficiency	B. any substance that provokes an immune response
_____ 3. helper T cells	C. an endocrine gland located near the base of the neck
_____ 4. HIV	D. a medical condition characterized by a particular group of signs and symptoms
_____ 5. SLE	E. a type of white blood cells
_____ 6. lymphoma	F. a disease caused by antibodies attacking the normal tissues and organs of the body
_____ 7. antibody	G. a disease in which excess thyroid hormone is secreted

_____ 8. antigen   H. weakness in a person's immune system

_____ 9. Graves' disease   I. the malignant tumor of lymph nodes

_____ 10. thyroid   J. any protein present in the body that can identify and neutralize foreign substances

Ⅲ. **Translate the following Chinese sentences into English.**

1. 健康的免疫系统可以成功对抗各种可致病抗原及攻击人体的外源性异物。

2. 新合成的病毒可穿破垂死的辅助性 T 细胞，继续循环性感染杀死其他辅助性 T 细胞。

3. 重症联合免疫缺陷代表一组罕见的、有时可致命的先天性疾病，以机体少免疫应答或无免疫应答为特点。

4. 系统性红斑狼疮是一种抗体把自身组织器官当作外源性物质进行攻击的疾病。

5. 鉴于非霍奇金淋巴瘤的治愈率低于霍奇金淋巴瘤，因此，早期发现和治疗至关重要。

Ⅳ. **Think critically and then answer the following questions.**

1. Explain why the lymphatic system is a one-way system, whereas the blood vascular system is a two-way system.

2. Mr. Zhang's daughter was born without a thymus gland. Immediate plans were made for a thymus transplantation to be performed. In the meantime, she was placed in strict isolation. For what reason was she placed in isolation?

Medicine in China

More Efforts Urged to Curb HIV/AIDS

While China's HIV/AIDS containment remains stable though challenging, officials and experts have called for intensified efforts to prevent transmission of HIV/AIDS, including raising wider awareness and resorting to early intervention methods for high-risk groups.

The country registered over 1.05 million people living with HIV and 351,000 cumulative deaths by the end of 2020, according to an article published on China CDC Weekly, an academic platform established by the Chinese Center for Disease

Control and Prevention.

As the proportion of HIV transmission by injection drug users dropped from 25.2 percent in 2009 to less than 2.5 percent in 2020, transmissions through heterosexual and homosexual activities both increased. Men who have sex with men are at the highest risk of contracting the virus in China, and innovative interventions are needed to boost their awareness of using HIV medications and receiving prompt tests, the article said.

"Integrating social media with the distribution of self-test kits also holds promise to increase HIV testing coverage and case identification," said the article, which was written by Dr. He Na, an epidemiology professor at Fudan University's School of Public Health in Shanghai.

The article also said that promoting safe sex and awareness of HIV among young people remains a major challenge. Data previously released by health authorities showed that China reports around 3,000 new HIV infections among young students each year, with the average age becoming younger over the years. The article said that anonymous, urine-based HIV testing via vending machines should be "a power complement to current interventions that target at-risk students and promote HIV testing".

Peng Liyuan, wife of President Xi Jinping and the World Health Organization's goodwill ambassador for tuberculosis and HIV/AIDS, called on people from all walks of life in all countries to join hands and take action to strengthen the prevention and treatment of AIDS, in order to benefit all mankind and build a global community of health for all.

Exercises

Ⅰ. **Translate the underlined part into Chinese.**

Ⅱ. **Answer the following question.**

What can be done to reduce HIV infections among young students?

Chapter 13

Reproductive System

Pre-Reading Question

A saying goes like this, "Life is a flame that is always burning itself out, but it catches fire again every time a child is born." What can you infer from this saying?

Reading

Text A   Structure and Functions of the Reproductive System

Male Reproductive System

In the male reproductive system (Figure 13-1), **sperms** are produced in the testes located in the scrotum. Normal body temperature is too hot, which is lethal to sperms, so the testes are outside of the abdominal cavity where the temperature is about 2°C lower.[1] If a man takes too many long, very hot baths, this can reduce his sperm count. **Undescended** testes will cause **sterility** because their environment is too warm for sperm viability unless the problem can be surgically corrected. From there[2], sperms are transferred to the **epididymides**. Coiled tubules, also found within the scrotum, store sperms and are the site of the final maturation of sperms. In **ejaculation**, sperms are forced up into the **vasa deferentia**. From the epididymides, the vasa deferentia go up, around the front of, over the top of, and behind the bladder.

The ends of the vasa deferentia, behind and slightly under the bladder, are called the **ejaculatory** ducts. The **seminal vesicles** are also located behind the bladder. Their secretions are about 60% of the total volume of the semen and contain mucus, **amino** acids, and **fructose** as the main energy source for the sperm, and **prostaglandins** to stimulate female **uterine** contractions to move the semen up into the uterus. The seminal vesicles empty the semen into the ejaculatory ducts. The ejaculatory ducts then empty the semen into the urethra.

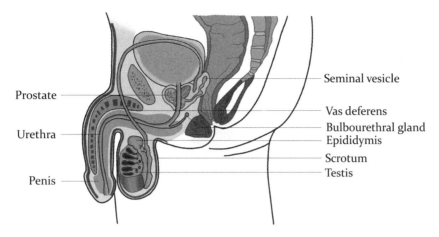

Figure 13-1   Structure of the male reproductive system

The initial **segment** of the urethra is surrounded by the prostate gland. The prostate is the largest of the accessory glands and puts its secretions directly into the urethra. These secretions are **alkaline** to buffer any residual urine, which tends to be **acidic**. The prostate needs a lot of **zinc** to function properly, and insufficient dietary zinc (as well as other causes) can lead to enlargement, which potentially can **constrict** the urethra to the point of interfering with urination.

The **bulbourethral** glands are a small pair of glands along the urethra below the prostate. Their fluid is secreted just before the **emission** of the semen; therefore, it is thought that this fluid may serve as a **lubricant** for inserting the penis into the **vagina**. However, because the volume of these secretions is very small, people are not totally sure of this function.

The urethra goes through the penis. In humans, the penis contains three **cylinders** of spongy, **erectile** tissue. During **arousal**, these become filled with blood from the arteries that supply them, and the pressure seals off the veins that drain these areas, causing an **erection**, which is necessary for the insertion of the penis into the woman's vagina.[3] The head of the penis, the **glans penis**, is very sensitive to stimulation.

Female Reproductive System

In the female reproductive system (Figure 13-2), **eggs** are produced in the ovaries. Within the ovary, a follicle consists of one **precursor** egg cell surrounded by special cells to nourish and protect it. A female typically has about 400,000 follicles/potential eggs, all formed before birth. Only several hundred of these eggs will actually ever be released during her reproductive years. Normally, after the **onset** of puberty, due to the stimulation of follicle-stimulating hormone (FSH), one egg per cycle matures and is released from its ovary. **Ovulation** is the release of mature eggs due to the stimulation of **luteinizing** hormone (LH), which then stimulates the remaining follicle cells to turn into a **corpus luteum** which then secretes progesterone to prepare the uterus for possible implantation. If an egg is not **fertilized** and does not implant, the corpus luteum disintegrates and when it stops producing progesterone, the lining of the uterus breaks down and is shed.

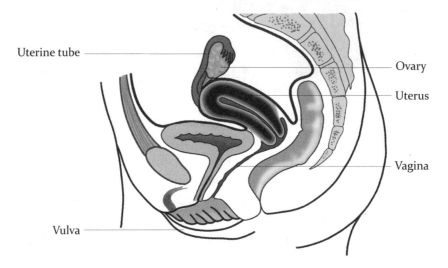

Uterine tube
Ovary
Uterus
Vagina
Vulva

Figure 13-2   Structure of the female reproductive system

Each egg is released into the abdominal cavity near the opening of one of the **oviducts**. Cilia in the oviduct set up currents that draw the egg in. If sperms are present in the oviduct, the egg will be fertilized near the far end of the oviduct and quickly finish **meiosis**, and the **embryo** will start to divide and grow as it travels to the uterus. The trip down the oviduct takes about a week as the cilia propel the fertilized egg or the embryo down to the uterus. During this time, progesterone secreted by the corpus luteum has been stimulating the **endometrium**, the lining of the uterus, to thicken in preparation for possible implantation.[4] When a growing embryo finally reaches the uterus, it will implant in this **nutritious** environment and begin to secrete its own hormones to maintain the endometrium. If the egg is not fertilized, it dies and disintegrates, and as the corpus luteum also disintegrates, its progesterone production falls, and the unneeded, built-up endometrium is shed. This process is called **menstruation**.

The uterus has thick muscular walls and is very small. In those who have never given birth, the uterus is only about 7 cm long by 4 to 5 cm wide, but it can expand to hold a baby of 4 kg. The endometrium has a rich capillary supply to bring food to any embryo that might implant there.

The bottom end of the uterus is called the **cervix**. The cervix secretes mucus, the consistency of which varies with the stages in her menstrual cycle.[5] At ovulation, the cervical mucus is clear, runny, and beneficial to sperms. During the post-ovulation period, the mucus gets thick and **pasty** to block sperms. If a woman becomes pregnant, the cervical mucus forms a plug to seal off the uterus and protect the developing baby.

The vagina is a relatively thin-walled chamber. It serves as a storage for sperms, and also serves as the birth canal. Unlike males, females have separate openings for the urinary and reproductive systems. These openings are covered externally by two sets of skin **folds**. The thinner, inner folds are the **labia minora** and the thicker, outer ones are the **labia majora**. The labia minora contain erectile tissue like that in the penis and thus change shape when the woman is sexually aroused. The opening around the **genital** area is called the **vestibule**. There is a membrane called the **hymen** that partially covers the opening of the vagina. This is torn by the woman's first sexual intercourse.

At the anterior end of the labia, under the **pubic** bone, is the **clitoris**, the female **equivalent** of the penis. This small structure contains erectile tissue and many nerve endings in a sensitive glans within a **prepuce** which totally encloses the glans, which is the most sensitive point for female sexual stimulation.

▶ Word Bank

sperm /spɜːm/ *n.* 精液；精子

sterility /stəˈrɪləti/ *n.* 不生育

epididymidis /ˌepɪˈdɪdɪmɪdɪs/ *n.* 附睾（复数为 epididymides）

ejaculation /ɪˌdʒækjʊˈleɪʃən/ *n.* 射精

vas deferens /ˈvæs ˈdefərens/ *n.* 输精管（复数为 vasa deferentia）

ejaculatory /ɪˈdʒækjʊˌlətərɪ/ *a.* 射精的；射出的

seminal /ˈsemɪnəl/ *a.* 种子的；精液的；生殖的

vesicle /ˈvesɪkl/ *n.* 泡；囊

fructose /ˈfrʲuktəʊz/ *n.* 果糖

uterine /ˈjuːtərɪn/ *a.* 子宫的

alkaline /ˈælkəlaɪn/ *a.* 碱的；碱性的

zinc /zɪŋk/ *n.* 锌

bulbourethral /ˌbʌlbəˈriːθrəl/ *a.* 尿道球部的

lubricant /ˈluːbrɪkənt/ *n.* 润滑剂

cylinder /ˈsɪlɪndə/ *n.* 圆筒；汽缸；圆柱体

arousal /əˈraʊzəl/ *n.* 激励；唤醒；激发

glans penis /glænz ˈpiːnɪs/ *n.* 龟头

precursor /priːˈkɜːsə/ *n.* 先驱；前任；前兆

ovulation /ˌɒvjʊˈleɪʃən/ *n.* 排卵

corpus luteum /ˈkɔːpəs luːˈtiːəm/ *n.* 黄体

undescended /ˌʌndɪˈsendɪd/ *a.*（睾丸）未降到阴囊的

amino /əˈmiːnəʊ/ *n.* 氨基

prostaglandin /ˌprɒstəˈɡlændɪn/ *n.* 前列腺素

segment /ˈseɡmənt/ *n.* 部分；段；节

acidic /əˈsɪdɪk/ *a.* 酸的；酸性的

constrict /kənˈstrɪkt/ *v.* 压缩；束紧；使收缩

emission /ɪˈmɪʃən/ *n.* 散发，排放

vagina /vəˈdʒaɪnə/ *n.* 阴道

erectile /ɪˈrektəl/ *a.* 可直立的；勃起的

erection /ɪˈrekʃən/ *n.* 勃起

egg /eɡ/ *n.* 卵子

onset /ˈɒnset/ *n.* 开始；攻击，进攻

luteinize /ˈluːtiːɪnaɪz/ *v.* 黄体化

fertilize /ˈfɜːtɪlaɪz/ *v.* 受精

disintegrate /dɪsˈɪntɪgreɪt/ *v.* 瓦解，崩溃

meiosis /maɪˈəʊsɪs/ *n.* 细胞核减数分裂

endometrium /ˌendəʊˈmiːtrɪəm/ *n.* 子宫内膜

menstruation /ˌmenstrʊˈeɪʃən/ *n.* 月经；月经期间

pasty /ˈpæstɪ/ *a.* 浆糊的

labium minus /ˈleɪbɪəm ˈmaɪnəs/ 小阴唇（复数为 labia minora）

labium majus /ˈleɪbɪəm ˈmeɪdʒəs/ 大阴唇（复数为 labia majora）

genital /ˈdʒenɪtəl/ *a.* 生殖的；生殖器的

hymen /ˈhaɪmən/ *n.* 处女膜

pubic /ˈpjuːbɪk/ *a.* 阴毛的；阴部的；耻骨的

equivalent /ɪˈkwɪvələnt/ *n.* 相等物

oviduct /ˈəʊvɪdʌkt/ *n.* 输卵管

embryo /ˈembrɪəʊ/ *n.* 胚胎；萌芽

nutritious /njʊˈtrɪʃəs/ *a.* 有营养的，滋养的

cervix /ˈsɜːvɪks/ *n.* 颈部；子宫颈

fold /fəʊld/ *n.* 折层；折痕，皱褶

vestibule /ˈvestɪbjuːl/ *n.* 阴道前庭

intercourse /ˈɪntəkɔːs/ *n.* 性交

clitoris /ˈklɪtərɪs/ *n.* 阴核；阴蒂

prepuce /ˈpriːpjuːs/ *n.* 阴茎包皮

▶ Notes

1. 该句中包含两个定语从句。第一个定语从句由 which 引导，其先行词是前面一整句话 Normal body temperature is too hot。第二个定语从句由 where 引导，其先行词是 abdominal cavity。

2. 此处 there 指的是 testes。

3. 该句较复杂，these 指前句中提到的 three cylinders of spongy 和 erectile tissue。arteries 后有一个 that 引导的定语从句来修饰它。veins 后也有一个 that 引导的定语从句。causing 为现在分词作结果状语；which 引导的非限定性定语从句修饰的先行词为 erection。

4. 该句中 secreted by the corpus luteum 为过去分词短语充当定语，修饰 progesterone。has been stimulating 为谓语，the lining of the uterus 是 endometrium 的同位语，to thicken in preparation for possible implantation 为不定式短语作目的状语。

5. 该句中 the consistency of which varies with the stages in her menstrual cycle 是由 which 引导的非限定性定语从句，其先行词是 mucus。

Exercises

Ⅰ. Choose the best answer to each of the following questions.

1. Where are the sperms stored?
   A. The scrotum. B. The epididymis.
   C. The coiled tubules. D. The vasa deferentia.

2. What is the best temperature for sperm viability?
   A. 34.5 ℃. B. 36.5 ℃.

C. 38 ℃. 　　　　　　　　　　　　　D. 28 ℃.

3.　Which sequence best represents the path taken by sperms from the site of origin to the exterior?

　　A. Testes, epididymis, vasa deferentia, coiled tubules, ejaculatory ducts, urethra.

　　B. Testes, vasa deferentia, coiled tubules, epididymides, ejaculatory ducts, urethra.

　　C. Testes, vasa deferentia, epididymides, coiled tubules, ejaculatory ducts, urethra.

　　D. Testes, coiled tubules, epididymides, vasa deferentia, ejaculatory ducts, urethra.

4.　Which structure is the male urethra encircled by?

　　A. The epididymides.　　　　　　　B. The scrotum.

　　C. The prostate.　　　　　　　　　D. The seminal vesicle.

5.　What can be said about bulbourethral glands?

　　A. They secrete lubricant before ejaculation.

　　B. They secrete fluid during ejaculation.

　　C. They secrete fluid before ejaculation.

　　D. They secrete the semen during ejaculation.

6.　Which of the following can best describe the relationship between the urethra and the penis?

　　A. The urethra has an opening in the penis.

　　B. The urethra goes through the penis.

　　C. The urethra and the penis go along with each other.

　　D. The urethra is filled with blood, which helps the penis erect.

7.　What does the corpus luteum secrete?

　　A. Follicle.

　　B. Follicle-stimulating hormone.

　　C. Luteinizing hormone.

　　D. Progesterone.

8.　Fertilization normally occurs in the _____.

　　A. oviduct　　　　　　　　　　　　B. vagina

　　C. uterus　　　　　　　　　　　　 D. ovaries

9.　The opening of the uterus to the vagina is called _____.

　　A. the vestibule　　　　　　　　　B. the endometrium

　　C. the cervix　　　　　　　　　　 D. the capillary

10. Which of the following is the female equivalent of penis?
   A. The labia minora.   B. The labia majora.
   C. The hymen.   D. The clitoris.

Ⅱ. **Group the following terms into the major categories they belong to.**

sperm, egg, ovary, scrotum, follicle-stimulating hormone, epididymides, cervix, bulbourethral gland, menstruation, vagina, vasa deferentia, testes, prostate gland

Male reproductive system: _____

_____

Female reproductive system: _____

_____

Ⅲ. **Fill in each blank in the following paragraph with a word in the box. Change the form of words if necessary.**

productive	oviduct	estrogen	cycle	sperm
ovulation	puberty	reproductive	sex	menstruation
structure	ovary	size	period	pituitary

Most species have two 1_____: male and female. Each sex has its own unique 2_____ system. They are different in shape and 3_____, but both are specifically designed to produce, nourish, and transport either the egg or 4_____. When a baby girl is born, her 5_____ contain hundreds of thousands of eggs, which remain inactive until puberty begins. At puberty, the 6_____ gland, located in the central part of the brain, starts making hormones that stimulate the ovaries to produce female sex hormones, including 7_____. The secretion of these hormones causes a girl to develop into a sexually mature woman. Toward the end of puberty, the girl begins to release eggs as part of a monthly period called the menstrual 8_____. Approximately once a month, during 9_____, an ovary sends a tiny egg into one of the 10_____.

Ⅳ. **Translate the following English sentences into Chinese.**

1. Normal body temperature is too hot, which is lethal to sperms, so the testes are outside of the abdominal cavity where the temperature is about 2°C lower.

2. Their secretions are about 60% of the total volume of the semen and contain mucus, amino acids, and fructose as the main energy source for the sperm, and prostaglandins to stimulate female uterine contractions to move the semen up into the uterus.

3. Insufficient dietary zinc (as well as other causes) can lead to enlargement, which potentially can constrict the urethra to the point of interfering with urination.

4. Within the ovary, a follicle consists of one precursor egg cell surrounded by special cells to nourish and protect it.

5. If a woman becomes pregnant, the cervical mucus forms a plug to seal off the uterus and protect the developing baby.

Ⅴ. **Write a 50-word summary of the mechanism of the menstruation cycle.**

Reading

Text B   Diseases of the Reproductive System and Their Treatment

Many parts of the male and female reproductive systems can be affected by cancer. In females, cancer can attack the uterus, ovaries, breast and cervix, and other organs. Males can develop prostate, **testicular**, and **penile** cancers.

Both genders can develop sexually transmitted diseases, including genital **herpes**, **gonorrhea**, and **syphilis**. AIDS, a disease of the immune system, is not **exclusively** transmitted through sexual contact; sexual activity is one of the ways that the human immunodeficiency virus (HIV) is spread. Roughly sexual transmission is responsible for about 80% of the world's HIV infections. Mother-to-child transmission of HIV during pregnancy, delivery, or breast-feeding is the second leading mode of spread of HIV and causes roughly 600,000 new infections annually. Transmission through injection drug use continues to play a major role in HIV epidemics in several regions of the world, particularly Eastern Europe and Asia.

Genital human **papillomavirus** (HPV) is the most common sexually transmitted infection. Most sexually active people in the United States, male and female, will have HPV at some time in their lives. In most people, it causes no problems, but it can result in cervical cancer and genital **warts** in women and it can cause penile and anal cancer and genital warts in men.

For females, **vaginitis** is a common disorder, which is caused by a **yeast** fungus in the vagina. Yeast is commonly present on normal human skin and in areas of **moisture**, such as the mouth and vagina. In fact, it is estimated that between 20% and 50% of healthy women normally carry yeast in the vaginal area. The specific type of fungus most commonly responsible for vaginitis is **Candida albicans**. Yeast vaginitis is characterized by itching, burning, **soreness**, pain during intercourse and/or urination and vaginal discharge. It can be spread to a male or female partner. Symptoms of a yeast infection in a man are itching and irritation of the penis after sexual contact with an infected woman. This disease can be treated with **antifungal** medications applied to the affected area or taken by mouth.

Endometriosis is a condition involving **colonization** of the abdominal/pelvic cavity with patches of endometrial tissue. If endometrial tissue flushes up the uterine tube during menstruation and spills into the abdomen, the clots of endometrial tissue can attach to abdominal organs such as the bladder, rectum, and intestinal loops and then cycle along with the uterus in response to monthly changes in **ovarian** hormones.

A major symptom of endometriosis is recurring pelvic pain. The pain can range from mild to severe cramping or stabbing pain that occurs on both sides of the pelvis, in the lower back and **rectal** area, and even down the legs. The amount of pain a woman feels correlates poorly with the extent or stage of endometriosis. Some women have little or no pain despite having extensive endometriosis or endometriosis with scarring, while other women may have severe pain even though they have only a few small areas of endometriosis.

While there is no cure for endometriosis, there are two types of interventions: treatment of pain and treatment of **infertility**. In many women menopause (natural or surgical) will relieve the process. In patients in the reproductive years, endometriosis is merely managed: the goal is to provide pain relief, restrict the progression of the process, and restore or preserve fertility. In younger women with unfulfilled reproductive potential, surgical treatment attempts to remove endometrial tissue and preserve the ovaries without damaging normal tissue.

Pelvic inflammatory disease is a condition where bacteria make their way up the vagina through the uterus and **traverse** the uterine tubes which open into the abdominal cavity. The disease can be asymptomatic or life-threatening. Patients should be treated **empirically**, even if they present with few symptoms. Most women can be treated successfully as outpatients with a single dose of a **parenteral**

cephalosporin plus oral **doxycycline**, with or without oral **metronidazole**. Delays in treatment may be serious, leading to chronic pelvic pain, **ectopic** pregnancy, and infertility. Hospitalization and parenteral treatment are recommended if the patient is pregnant, has an HIV infection, does not respond to oral medication, or is severely ill.

Infertility is defined as a couple's inability to **conceive** after one year of regular intercourse. In women, infertility is defined as a disorder of the reproductive system that hinders the body's ability to ovulate, conceive, or carry an infant to term[1]. In males, infertility is a condition in which they produce no sperm cells (**azoospermia**) or too few sperm cells (**oligospermia**[2]), or if their sperm cells are abnormal or die before they can reach the egg. Chronic problems with ejaculation also contribute to male infertility. In rare cases, infertility in men is caused by an inherited condition, such as cystic fibrosis or chromosomal abnormalities.

Men can also experience **epididymitis**, which is an inflammation of the epididymis. Epididymitis is usually caused by the spread of a bacterial infection from the urethra, prostate, or bladder. The most common infections that cause this condition in young **heterosexual** men are gonorrhea and **chlamydia**. In children and older men, **E. coli** and similar infections are much more common.

Another condition of the male reproductive system is **hypogonadism**, which occurs when the testicles do not produce enough testosterone. In boys, it causes impaired muscle and beard development and reduced height. In men, it can cause reduced body hair and beard, enlarged breasts, loss of muscle, and sexual difficulties. Hypogonadism is most often treated with testosterone replacement therapy in patients who are not trying to conceive. Commonly used testosterone replacement therapies include using a **patch** or **gel**, injections, or **pellets** through the skin.

▶ Word Bank

testicular /tes'tıkjʊlə/ *a.* 睾丸的

herpes /'hɜːpiːz/ *n.* 疱疹

syphilis /'sıfılıs/ *n.* 梅毒

papillomavirus /ˌpæpɪ'ləʊməˌvaɪrəs/ *n.* 乳头瘤病毒

wart /wɔːt/ *n.* 疣

yeast /jiːst/ *n.* 酵母

Candida albicans /'kændıdə 'ælbıkənz/ *n.* 白色念珠菌；白假丝酵母

soreness /'sɔːnıs/ *n.* 痛苦

endometriosis /ˌendəʊˌmiːtrɪ'əʊsıs/ *n.* 子宫内膜异位

colonization /ˌkɒlənaɪ'zeɪʃən/ *n.* 大量生长繁殖

penile /'piːnaɪl/ *a.* 阴茎的

gonorrhea /ˌgɒnə'riːə/ *n.* 淋病

exclusively /ık'skluːsıvlı/ *ad.* 专门地；排他地；仅仅

vaginitis /ˌvædʒə'naɪtıs/ *n.* 阴道炎

moisture /'mɔɪstʃə/ *n.* 湿度；水分；潮气

antifungal /ˌæntaɪ'fʌŋgəl/ *a.* 抗真菌的，杀真菌的

ovarian /əʊ'veərɪən/ *a.* 卵巢的

rectal /'rektəl/ *a.* 直肠的

infertility /ˌɪnfɜ:'tɪlɪtɪ/ *n.* 不孕；不育

traverse /trə'vɜ:s/ *v.* 横贯，穿越

empirically /ɪm'pɪrɪklɪ/ *ad.* 经验主义地

parenteral /pə'rentərəl/ *a.* 肠胃外的；不经肠道的

cephalosporin /ˌsefələʊ'spɔ:rɪn/ *n.* 头孢菌素

doxycycline /ˌdɒksɪ'saɪklɪn/ *n.* 多西环素

metronidazole /ˌmetrə'naɪdəzəʊl/ *n.* 灭滴灵，甲硝唑

ectopic /ek'tɒpɪk/ *a.* 异位的

conceive /kən'si:v/ *v.* 怀孕

azoospermia /əˈzu:spəmɪə/ *n.* 无精症

oligospermia /ˌɒlɪɡə'spəmɪə/ *n.* 少精症

epididymitis /ˌepɪˌdɪdɪ'maɪtɪs/ *n.* 附睾炎

heterosexual /ˌhetərə'sekʃʊəl/ *a.* 异性恋的

chlamydia /klə'mɪdɪə/ *n.* 衣原体；衣原体疾病

E. coli /ˌi:'kəʊlɪ/ *n.* 大肠埃希氏菌；大肠杆菌（全称为 Escherichia coli）

hypogonadism /ˌhaɪpəʊ'ɡɒnæˌdɪzəm/ *n.* 性腺机能减退，生殖官能不良

patch /pætʃ/ *n.* 小片；膏药

gel /dʒel/ *n.* 凝胶；发胶

pellet /'pelɪt/ *n.* 小球；小药丸

▶ 注释 Notes

1. carry an infant to term 意为怀孕到足月，term 意为期限，以 term 为同根的衍生词有 preterm（早产儿）。

2. 在 oligospermia 一词中，构词成分 spermia 为 spermium 的复数，意为精子。oligo- 为前缀，表示"少"的意思，如：oliguria（少尿）、oligoxylose（低聚木糖）等。

Exercises

Ⅰ. **For each of the following statements, write "T" if the statement is true and "F" if the statement is false in the blank.**

_____ 1. Sexual activity is a major way for HIV to spread.

_____ 2. Although HPV may be carried by both males and females, it only affects females.

_____ 3. Candida albicans may cause vaginitis in women and penis irritation in men.

_____ 4. Endometrial tissue may grow in organs in the abdominal cavity.

_____ 5. For patients in their reproductive years, endometriosis cannot be treated.

_____ 6. For elderly women, surgery can be performed to remove endometrial tissue to preserve the ovaries.

_____ 7. Women with asymptomatic pelvic inflammatory disease do not need treatment.

_____ 8. Both males and females may suffer from infertility.

_____ 9. Epididymitis can be caused by bacteria, viruses, or other microorganisms.

_____ 10. Male patients with hypogonadism may present female physical traits.

Ⅱ. **Match each term in Column A with its correct description in Column B. Write the corresponding letter in the blank.**

Column A	Column B
_____ 1. asymptomatic	A. a sexually transmitted infection caused by HPV
_____ 2. azoospermia	B. yeast fungus infection of the vagina
_____ 3. endometriosis	C. having no symptoms
_____ 4. epididymitis	D. a condition caused by bacteria entering the pelvic cavity
_____ 5. genital warts	E. inability to produce offspring
_____ 6. infertility	F. colonization of endometrial tissue in other organs
_____ 7. oligospermia	G. a condition where a male produces no sperm cells
_____ 8. pelvic inflammation	H. a male hormone
_____ 9. testosterone	I. a condition where a male produces too few sperm cells
_____ 10. vaginitis	J. inflammation of the epididymis

Ⅲ. **Translate the following Chinese sentences into English.**

1. 母婴传播是艾滋病的第二大传播方式，每年大约引发 60 万例新增病例。

2. 酵母菌性阴道炎的主要表现是瘙痒、灼痛、酸痛、性交痛或排尿痛以及阴道分泌物增多。

3. 可能是盆腔两侧、下背部和直肠区甚至腿部的轻微疼痛，也可能是严重绞痛或刺痛。

4. 对于具有生育需求的年轻女性，手术治疗的目的是切除子宫内膜组织，保留卵巢，但不破坏正常组织。

5. 女性不育是生殖系统疾病，身体不能排卵、怀孕，或者孕期流产。

Ⅳ. **Think critically and then answer the following questions.**

1. A 1-year-old boy was admitted to hospital because examinations indicated that he had no penis, but the testicular tissue was present. Besides, X-ray showed that he had ovaries. If you were the doctor, what management would you suggest?

2. A couple had no child after two years of regular intercourse, and their condition was diagnosed as infertility. What might be the causes of their condition?

Medicine in China

Measures to Increase Births Expected to Be Introduced

A key report delivered to the 20th National Congress of the Communist Party of China held in October 2022 stresses that the country will establish a policy system to boost birthrates and bring down the costs of pregnancy and childbirth, child rearing, and schooling.

The annual number of new births in China has slipped about 40 percent in the past five years. Data shows that the Chinese mainland recorded 9.56 million newborns in 2022, compared with 12 million in 2020 and 17.86 million in 2016. Experts said the falling number of new births is a major factor contributing to the historic population decline recorded in 2022. China's fertility rate dropped below the replacement level of 2.1—the minimum threshold for keeping a stable population—in 1992 and has remained at a low level since. Official data show that in 2020 the rate fell to 1.3.

To tackle falling birthrates and a looming decline in population, the central leadership released a decision in 2021 to allow all couples to have three children, up from two, and to roll out supportive policies, such as extending maternity leave and issuing fertility subsidies.

"The policy shift has not yielded expected outcomes thus far. So the report signals that boosting fertility remains the core of China's population work in the future, and systematic measures surrounding fertility should be established," said Lu Jiehua, a sociology professor at Peking University and vice-president of the China Population Association.

Lu added favorable policies, such as longer maternity or paternity leave and subsidies, should not only target families pondering whether to have a third child but also those planning to have their first.

Exercises

Ⅰ. **Translate the underlined part into Chinese.**

Ⅱ. **Answer the following question.**

What measures can be taken to increase births in China?

Chapter 14

Integumentary System

Pre-Reading Question

What is the meaning of "Beauty is only skin deep?" Do you know the thickness of skin?

Reading

Text A Anatomy and Functions of the Integumentary System

The skin covers the entire external surface of the human body and is the principal site of interaction with the surrounding world. It serves as a protective barrier that **interfaces** with a sometimes hostile environment. It is also very involved in maintaining the proper temperature for the body to function well. It gathers sensory information from the environment and plays an active role in the immune system, protecting us from diseases. The **integument** consists of two mutually dependent layers, the epidermis, and **dermis**, which rest on a **fatty** subcutaneous layer, the **hypodermis** (Figure 14-1).

Epidermis

The epidermis is the outer layer of skin that covers almost the entire body surface. The epidermis protects the deeper and thicker dermis layer of the skin. The thickness of the epidermis varies in different types of skin. It is the thinnest on the eyelids at 0.05 mm and the thickest on the **palms** and **soles** at 1.5 mm. The epidermis does not contain any blood vessels. The cells of the epidermis receive all of their nutrients via **diffusion** of fluids from the dermis.

The epidermis is made of several specialized types of cells. Almost 90% of the epidermis is made of cells known as **keratinocytes**[1]. Keratinocytes develop from **stem** cells at the base of the epidermis, and produce and store the protein **keratin**. Keratin makes the keratinocytes very tough, **scaly**, and **water-resistant**. About

8% of epidermal cells are **melanocytes**, which form the second most numerous cell type in the epidermis. Melanocytes produce the pigment **melanin** to protect the skin from **ultraviolet** radiation and **sunburn**. **Langerhans cells** make up just over 1% of all epidermal cells. The role of Langerhans cells is to detect and fight pathogens that attempt to enter the body through the skin. Finally, **Merkel cells** make up less than 1% of all epidermal cells but have an important function in sensing touch. Merkel cells form a disk along the deepest edge of the epidermis where they connect to nerve endings in the dermis to sense light touch.

The epidermis in most parts of the body is arranged into four distinct layers. In the **palmar** surface of the hands and **plantar** surface of the feet, the skin is thicker than that in the rest of the body and there is a fifth layer of the epidermis.

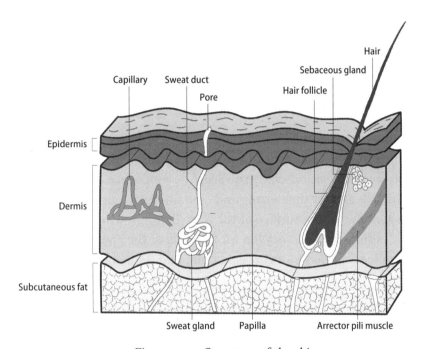

Figure 14-1 Structure of the skin

The bottom layer of the epidermis is the **stratum basale**, which contains the stem cells that reproduce to form all of the other cells of the epidermis. The cells of the stratum basale include **cuboidal** keratinocytes, melanocytes, and Merkel cells.

Superficial to the stratum basale is the stratum **spinosum** layer where Langerhans cells are found along with many rows of **spiny** keratinocytes.[2] The spines found here are cellular projections called **desmosomes** that form between keratinocytes to hold them together and resist friction.

Just superficial to the stratum spinosum is the stratum **granulosum**, where keratinocytes begin to produce **waxy lamellar** granules to **waterproof** the skin.

The keratinocytes in the stratum granulosum are so far removed from the dermis that they begin to die from lack of nutrients.

In the thick skin of the hands and feet, there is a layer of skin superficial to the stratum granulosum known as the stratum **lucidum**. The stratum lucidum is made of several rows of clear, dead keratinocytes that protect the underlying layers.

The outermost layer of skin is the stratum **corneum**. The stratum corneum is made of many rows of flattened, dead keratinocytes that protect the underlying layers. Dead keratinocytes are constantly shed from the surface of the stratum corneum and replaced by cells arriving from the deeper layers.

Dermis

The dermis is the deep layer of the skin found under the epidermis. The dermis is mostly made of dense irregular connective tissue along with nervous tissue, blood, and blood vessels. The dermis is much thicker than the epidermis and gives the skin its strength and elasticity. Within the dermis, there are two distinct regions: the **papillary** layer and the **reticular** layer.

The papillary layer is the superficial layer of the dermis that borders on the epidermis. The papillary layer contains many finger-like extensions called **dermal papillae** that protrude superficially towards the epidermis. The dermal papillae increase the surface area of the dermis and contain many nerves and blood vessels that are projected toward the surface of the skin. Blood flowing through the dermal papillae provides nutrients and oxygen for the cells of the epidermis. The nerves of the dermal papillae are used to feel touch, pain, and temperature through the cells of the epidermis.

The deeper layer of the dermis, the reticular layer, is the thicker and tougher part of the dermis. The reticular layer is made of dense irregular connective tissue that contains many tough collagen and **stretchy elastin** fibers running in all directions to provide strength and elasticity to the skin. The reticular layer also contains blood vessels to support the skin cells and nerve tissue to sense pressure and pain in the skin.

Hypodermis

Deep to the dermis is a layer of loose connective tissue known as the hypodermis, or subcutaneous tissue. The hypodermis serves as the flexible connection between the skin and the underlying muscles and bones as well as a fat storage area. **Areolar** connective tissue in the hypodermis contains elastin and collagen fibers loosely arranged to allow the skin to stretch and move independently of its underlying structures. Fatty **adipose** tissue in the hypodermis stores energy in the form of **triglycerides**. Adipose also helps to insulate the body by trapping body heat produced by the underlying muscles.

▶ Word Bank

integumentary /ɪnˌtegjʊ'mentərɪ/ *a.* 外皮的；外壳的

integument /ɪn'tegjʊmənt/ *n.* 覆盖物；外皮

fatty /'fætɪ/ *a.* 脂肪的；含脂肪的

palm /pɑ:m/ *n.* 手掌

diffusion /dɪ'fju:ʒən/ *n.* 扩散；散布；传播

stem /stem/ *n.* 干；柄；茎

scaly /'skeɪlɪ/ *a.* 有鳞的；剥落的

melanocyte /'melənəsaɪt/ *n.* 黑色素细胞

ultraviolet /ˌʌltrə'vaɪələt/ *a.* 紫外线的

Langerhans cell /'læŋgəhæns sel/ 郎格尔汉细胞，表皮黑素细胞

Merkel cell /'məkəl sel/ 梅克尔细胞，触觉上皮细胞

plantar /'plæntə/ *a.* 跖的，足底的

cuboidal /kju:'bɔɪdəl/ *a.* 立方形的；骰子形的

spinosum /spaɪ'nəʊsʌm/ *a.* 棘的

desmosome /'dezməʊsəm/ *n.* 细胞桥粒

waxy /'wæksɪ/ *a.* 像蜡的；蜡色的；苍白的；光滑的

waterproof /'wɔ:təpru:f/ *v.* 防水

corneum /'kɔ:nɪəm/ *n.* 角质层

reticular /rɪ'tɪkjʊlə/ *a.* 网的；网状的；网状组织的

papilla /pə'pɪlə/ *n.* 乳头状突起（复数为 papillae）

elastin /ɪ'læstɪn/ *n.* 弹力素，弹性蛋白

adipose /'ædɪpəʊs/ *a.* 脂肪的；多脂肪的

interface /'ɪntəfeɪs/ *v.* 联系；相互作用；界面

dermis /'dɜ:mɪs/ *n.* 真皮

hypodermis /ˌhaɪpəʊ'dɜ:mɪs/ *n.* 皮下组织

sole /səʊl/ *n.* 脚掌

keratinocyte /'kerətɪnəˌsaɪt/ *n.* 角质形成细胞

keratin /'kerətɪn/ *n.* 角蛋白，角质素

water-resistant /'wɔ:tə rɪ'zɪstənt/ *a.* 防水的

melanin /'melənɪn/ *n.* 黑色素

sunburn /'sʌnbɜ:n/ *n.* 日灼，晒伤

palmar /'pælmə/ *a.* 手掌的，掌中的

stratum basale 基底层

superficial /ˌsu:pə'fɪʃəl/ *a.* 表面的；肤浅的

spiny /'spaɪnɪ/ *a.* 多刺的；困难的

granulosum /ˌgrænjʊ'ləʊsəm/ *a.* 颗粒的

lamellar /lə'melə/ *a.* 层状的；层式的

lucidum /'lu:si:dəm/ *a.* 透明的；清明的

papillary /'pæpɪlərɪ/ *a.* 乳突的；乳头状突起的

dermal /'dɜ:məl/ *a.* 皮肤的；真皮的

stretchy /'stretʃɪ/ *a.* 伸长的；有弹性的

areolar /ə'reəʊlə/ *a.* 网隙的；晕的

triglyceride /traɪ'glɪsəraɪd/ *n.* 甘油三酯

▶ Notes

1. keratinocytes 为角质形成细胞。此词中 -cyte 为词尾成分，意为细胞，keratin/o 为构词成分，意为角蛋白。

2. 该句为倒装句，主语为 the stratum spinosum layer，将表语 superficial to stratum basale 提到句首，一方面是为了强调棘层与基底层的位置关系，另一方面是因为主语连同其定语从句过长。类似的结构还有下一段的首句。

Exercises

Ⅰ. **Choose the best answer to each of the following questions.**

1. Why can the integumentary system protect the human body?
   A. Because it is the largest organ of the human body.
   B. Because it maintains body temperature.
   C. Because it immunizes the human body against diseases.
   D. Because it covers the external surface of the human body.

2. What is the function of Langerhans cells?
   A. Detecting and fighting pathogens.
   B. Sensing touch.
   C. Producing and storing the protein keratin.
   D. Producing the pigment melanin.

3. What is the relationship between epidermis and dermis?
   A. Epidermis is dependent on the dermis.
   B. Dermis is dependent on the epidermis.
   C. Epidermis provides nutrients for the dermis.
   D. Dermis provides nutrients for the epidermis.

4. Which of the following cells account for the largest proportion of the epidermis?
   A. Keratinocytes.   B. Stem cells.
   C. Langerhans cells.   D. Merkel cells.

5. What is the function of melanocytes?
   A. Producing and storing the protein keratin.
   B. Producing the pigment melanin.
   C. Detecting and fighting pathogens.
   D. Gathering sensory information.

6. What is the correct order for the layers of the epidermis from the innermost layer to the outermost layer?
   A. Tratum basale, stratum granulosum, stratum spinosum, stratum corneum.
   B. Stratum corneum, stratum spinosum, stratum basale, stratum granulosum.
   C. Stratum basale, stratum spinosum, stratum granulosum, stratum corneum.
   D. Stratum corneum, stratum basale, stratum spinosum, stratum granulosum.

7. Why is the stratum lucidum found in the thick skin of hands and feet?
   A. Because it is the fifth layer of the epidermis.

B. Because it is the thickest layer of the epidermis.

C. Because it is superficial to the stratum granulosum.

D. Because it can protect the underlying layers.

8. Which of the following is true about the dermal papillae?

A. They protrude towards the dermis.

B. They increase the surface area of the epidermis.

C. They contain nerves and blood vessels.

D. They provide nutrients and oxygen for cells of the dermis.

9. What is the function of the nerve tissue in the reticular layer?

A. Feeling pain and touch.

B. Feeling touch and temperature.

C. Feeling pain and pressure.

D. Feeling touch and pressure.

10. Why can the skin stretch and move independently of its underlying structures?

A. Because the hypodermis contains elastin and collagen.

B. Because the dermis contains collagen fibers.

C. Because the epidermis contains fat.

D. Because the hypodermis contains muscle.

Ⅱ. **Fill in each blank in the following paragraph with a word in the box. Change the form of words if necessary.**

aging	body	base	dermis	exposure
facial	granule	keratinocyte	melanocyte	melanosome
surface	pigment	radiation	trunk	stratum

The innermost layer of the epidermis which lies adjacent to the 1_____ comprises mainly dividing and non-dividing keratinocytes. As 2_____ divide and differentiate, they move from this deeper layer to the 3_____. Making up a small portion of the basal cell population is the pigment (melanin)-producing 4_____. The dendritic processes of these cells stretch between relatively large numbers of neighboring keratinocytes. Melanin accumulates in 5_____ that are transferred to the adjacent keratinocytes where they remain as 6_____. The melanin 7_____ provides protection against ultraviolet radiation; chronic 8_____ to light increases the ratio of melanocytes to keratinocytes, so more are found in the

9 _____ skin than on the lower back and a greater number on the outer arm than on the inner arm. 10 _____ diminishes the melanocyte population.

Ⅲ. Translate the following English sentences into Chinese.

1. The skin gathers sensory information from the environment and plays an active role in the immune system protecting us from diseases.

2. About 8% of epidermal cells are melanocytes, which form the second most numerous cell type in the epidermis.

3. The bottom layer of the epidermis is the stratum basale, which contains the stem cells that reproduce to form all of the other cells of the epidermis.

4. The dermal papillae increase the surface area of the dermis and contain many nerves and blood vessels that are projected toward the surface of the skin.

5. The hypodermis serves as the flexible connection between the skin and the underlying muscles and bones as well as a fat storage area.

Ⅳ. Write a 100-word summary of the layers and functions of the skin.

Reading

Text B   Diseases of the Integumentary System and Their Treatment

The skin, which is the largest organ in the body, is a tough, **resilient** barrier that covers the body and **shields** the muscle compartment and internal structures. It is composed of an outer epidermis of **ectodermal** origin and an underlying dermis of **mesenchymal** origin. The structure of the skin varies considerably from one area of the body to another, including changes in the thickness of its components and in its specialized structures of epithelial origin (e.g., hair, nails, sweat glands, and **sebaceous** glands). The skin is commonly affected by systemic diseases, and it is also the location of many diseases limited to the skin. It is often damaged by external stimuli such as radiation, sunlight, **toxins**, irritants, **allergens**, and infectious agents.

Nummular dermatitis occurs most frequently in patients who are in their 50s to 60s and is usually associated with significant dryness of the skin (**xerosis**). Both sexes are affected; in **temperate** climates, this condition is most frequently seen in winter. The condition appears to be more frequent among Asians. The origin of nummular dermatitis is unclear, although xerosis plays a significant role in its pathogenesis. Patients usually present with **pruritic**, coin-shaped, and **erythematous** patches with some **scales** and occasionally with **pinhead-sized vesicles**. Lesions may be **excoriated** and **lichenified**, such as thickened skin with **accentuation** of skin **markings**. Legs and arms are the commonly affected sites, although lesions can also occur on the trunk. All patients should be educated about the care of dry skin, such as the use of **emollients** and **moisturizing** soaps and **avoidance** of long, hot showers. **Topical** corticosteroid **ointments** are helpful for active lesions, and oral **antihistamines**[1] are useful for **pruritus**. In severe cases, narrow-band ultraviolet B (NB-UVB) **phototherapy**, **psoralen** combined with UVA (PUVA), or a short course of oral corticosteroids are beneficial.

Dyshidrosis appears as deep-seated, pinhead-sized vesicles, most commonly along the sides of the fingers. Occasionally, the palms and soles may also be involved. Lesions are usually pruritic, associated with xerosis of the surrounding skin. **Fissuring** of the tip and the sides of the fingers frequently occurs. Dyshidrosis is seen in individuals who wash their hands frequently, such as health care and restaurant workers and mothers of young infants. Treatment follows a **sequential** order: minimizing hand washing, liberal use of over-the-counter emollients, and topical corticosteroid ointments.

Atopic dermatitis is most commonly seen among young children, but severe cases persist into adulthood. The **prevalence** has been estimated at between 15% and 23%. In more than 80% of the patients, the disease starts before the age of 5 years. Patients usually present with xerosis, erythematous scaly patches, small vesicles, **excoriations**, **crusting**, and, not infrequently, **impetiginization**. With chronic **scratching** and rubbing, **hyperpigmentation**[2] and **lichenification** occur. Commonly affected sites include the **periorbital** area and flexor areas such as the neck, **antecubital fossa**, and **popliteal** fossa. In severe cases, the entire skin surface may be affected. Diagnosis is made by the typical **morphologic** features and by the distribution of the lesions, as well as by a family and personal history of **atopy**. The therapeutic ladder consists of the following: (1) over-the-counter emollients; (2) topical corticosteroid ointments, or topical **calcineurin** inhibitors. The U.S. Food and Drug Administration has warned of the potential association of the latter with the development of malignant disease; therefore, patients should be cautious of continuous prolonged use; (3) oral antihistamines; (4) NB-UVB phototherapy; and (5) PUVA. In patients with prolonged cases, oral prednisone, **cyclosporine**, and **mycophenolate mofetil** have been successful.

Seborrheic dermatitis is a common condition that occurs as erythematous patches with fine, **greasy**-appearing scales, most commonly on the **malar** area, **midforehead**, **midchest**, and **scalp**. This condition is common in patients with human immunodeficiency virus (HIV) infection. The diagnosis can usually be made on clinical grounds alone. Topical corticosteroids can rapidly reduce inflammation; then topical **ketoconazole** cream twice daily as needed is safe for long-term treatment.

Allergic contact dermatitis and irritant contact dermatitis are induced by exogenous agents. Allergic contact dermatitis is a delayed **hypersensitivity** response to external allergens, whereas irritant contact dermatitis is a **nonspecific** toxic response to contact irritants. In both conditions, lesions occur in the exposed area, but in patients with severe cases, **nonexposed** areas may also have milder lesions. In allergic contact dermatitis, patients present with pruritic erythematous **papules** followed by vesicles. Lesions are relieved with fine scales. **Postinflammatory** hyperpigmentation may be observed, especially in dark-skinned individuals. Irritant contact dermatitis manifests with lesions morphologically similar to those of allergic contact dermatitis, but usually associated with a burning **sensation** rather than with pruritus. Postinflammatory hyperpigmentation is frequently observed. Management includes identification and removal of the offending agent, as well as symptomatic treatments such as topical corticosteroids and oral antihistamines.

Whatever the disease, the goal of the therapy is to improve the skin condition with the least toxic and most specific approach. Because many treatments or medications can be applied directly to the skin, the option of topical therapy is attractive for treating many **dermatologic** diseases. However, many diseases require systemic therapies, particularly when patients have widespread involvement of the skin or a disease that cannot be improved with topical therapy. Therapies work by improving barrier function, removing scale, altering inflammation in the skin, altering blood flow, providing **antimicrobial** effects, or affecting **proliferating** cells.

▶ **Word Bank**

resilient /rɪ'zɪlɪənt/ *a.* 适应力强的；有弹力的   shield /ʃiːld/ *v.* 保护，庇护

ectodermal /ˌektəʊ'dɜːməl/ *a.* 外胚层的

mesenchymal /mes'eŋkɪməl/ *a.* 间叶细胞的；由间叶细胞组成的；间叶细胞样的

sebaceous/sɪ'beɪʃəs/ *a.* 脂肪的；似脂肪的；分泌油脂或皮脂的

toxin /'tɒksɪn/ *n.* 毒素，毒质   allergen /'ælədʒən/ *n.* 过敏原

nummular/'nʌmjʊlə/ *a.* 硬币形的；圆形的   dermatitis /ˌdɜːmə'taɪtɪs/ *n.* 皮肤炎

xerosis /zɪə'rəʊsɪs/ *n.* 干燥病   temperate /'tempərət/ *a.* 温和的；适度的；有节制的

pruritic /prʊ'rɪtɪk/ *a.* 痒的；瘙痒症的   erythematous /ˌerɪ'θiːmətəs/ *a.* 红斑状的

scale /skeɪl/ *n.* 鳞片，鳞状物   pinhead-sized /'pɪnhed 'saɪzd/ *a.* 针头大小的

excoriate /ɪeks'kɔːrɪeɪt/ *v.* 撕去皮   lichenified /laɪ'kenɪfaɪd/ *a.* 苔藓样变的，苔藓化的

accentuation /əkˌsentʃʊ'eɪʃən/ *n.* 强调；加强   marking /'mɑːkɪŋ/ *n.* 标志；斑纹

emollient /ɪ'mɒlɪənt/ n. 润肤剂

moisturize /'mɔɪstʃəraɪz/ v. 使湿润

avoidance /ə'vɔɪdəns/ n. 逃避，避免

topical /'tɒpɪkəl/ a. 局部的

ointment /'ɔɪntmənt/ n. 药膏；软膏

antihistamine /ˌæntɪ'hɪstəmiːn/ n. 抗组胺剂

pruritus /prʊ'raɪtəs/ n. 瘙痒

phototherapy /ˌfəʊtəʊ'θerəpɪ/ n. 光线疗法

psoralen /'sɔːrələn/ n. 补骨脂素

dyshidrosis /dɪs'haɪdrəʊsɪs/ n. 出汗障碍，出汗不良症

fissuring /'fɪʃərɪŋ/ n. 裂隙

sequential /sɪ'kwenʃəl/ a. 连续的

atopic /eɪ'tɒpɪk/ a. 异位的；遗传性过敏症的

prevalence /'prevələns/ n. 传播；流行，普及

excoriation /ˌekskɔːrɪ'eɪʃən/ n. 剥皮；抓痕

crusting /'krʌstɪŋ/ n. 结壳

impetiginization /ˌɪmpɪtɪˌdʒɪnɪ'zeɪʃən/ n. 脓疱化

scratching /'skrætʃɪŋ/ n. 刮擦

hyperpigmentation /ˌhaɪpəˌpɪgmen'teɪʃən/ n. 着色过度，色素沉着过度

lichenification /ˌlaɪkeˌnɪfɪ'keɪʃən/ n. 苔藓样硬化；苔藓样硬化斑

periorbital /ˌperɪ'ɔːbɪtəl/ a. 眶周的；眶骨膜的

antecubital /ˌæntɪ'kjuːbɪtəl/ a. 肘前的

fossa /'fɒsə/ n. 小窝；沟

popliteal /pɒp'lɪtɪəl/ a. 腿弯部的；膝后窝的

morphologic /ˌmɔːfə'lɒdʒɪk/ a. 形态学的

atopy /'ætəpɪ/ n. 异位性；特异反应性，特应性

calcineurin /kæl'saɪnjʊərɪn/ n. 钙调磷酸酶

cyclosporine /ˌsaɪkləʊ'spɔːriːn/ n. 环孢霉素

mycophenolate mofetil /ˌmaɪkɒ'fɪnəleɪt 'məʊvɪtɪl/ n. 麦考酚酸吗乙酯；麦考酚酸莫酯

seborrheic /ˌsebə'riːɪk/ a. 皮脂溢的

greasy /'griːsɪ/ a. 油腻的

malar /'meɪlə/ a. 颊的

midforehead /mɪd'fɔːhed/ n. 前额中部

midchest /mɪd'tʃest/ n. 胸部中间

scalp /skælp/ n. 头皮

ketoconazole /ˌkɪtəʊ'kəʊnəˌzəʊl/ n. 甲酮康唑

hypersensitivity /ˌhaɪpəˌsensə'tɪvətɪ/ n. 过敏症；超敏反应

nonspecific /ˌnɒnspɪ'sɪfɪk/ a. 非特异性的

nonexposed /ˌnɒnɪks'pəʊzd/ a. 未接触的；未暴露的

papule /'pæpjuːl/ n. 丘疹；小突起

postinflammatory /ˌpəʊstɪn'flæmətərɪ/ a. 炎症后的

sensation /sen'seɪʃən/ n. 感觉

dermatologic /ˌdɜːmətə'lɒdʒɪk/ a. 皮肤病学的

antimicrobial /ˌæntaɪmaɪ'krəʊbɪəl/ a. 抗菌的，抗微生物的

proliferate /prə'lɪfəreɪt/ v. 繁殖，增生

▶ Notes

1.　antihistamine 为抗组胺剂，anti- 为前缀，表示反对、排斥之意；histamine 为组织胺。又如：antioxidant（抗氧化物）。

2.　hyperpigmentation 为色素沉着过度，hyper- 为前缀，表示超级、超过、超越、高于、过度之义；pigment 意为色素；-ation 为后缀，表示名词化。又如：hypersensitive（过度敏感的）。

Exercises

Ⅰ. **For each of the following statements, write "T" if the statement is true and "F" if the statement is false in the blank.**

_____ 1. Skin diseases can be systemic and topical.

_____ 2. The skin can be affected by many diseases as it is the largest organ of the body.

_____ 3. Nummular dermatitis occurs often in elderly Asians in winter.

_____ 4. Avoiding long, hot showers can relieve dyshidrosis.

_____ 5. Xerosis is a common symptom shared by nummular dermatitis and atopic dermatitis.

_____ 6. Dyshidrosis occurs more often in adults while atopic dermatitis occurs more often in children.

_____ 7. Topical use of ointments can cure mild dermatitis.

_____ 8. HIV infection often causes seborrheic dermatitis.

_____ 9. Contact dermatitis may be caused by allergens or irritants.

_____ 10. Severe dermatitis often requires systemic medications.

Ⅱ. **Match each term in Column A with its correct description in Column B. Write the corresponding letter in the blank.**

Column A	olumn B
_____ 1. atopic dermatitis	A. dryness of the skin
_____ 2. contact dermatitis	B. a condition often affecting the sides of fingers
_____ 3. dermatitis	C. a condition often affecting the neck and antecubital fossa
_____ 4. dyshidrosis	D. a condition that often occurs as red patches with fine, greasy scales
_____ 5. hyperpigmentation	E. treatment with strong light
_____ 6. lichenification	F. a condition where the melatnin pigment gathers abnormally

_____ 7. pathogenesis

G. a condition where the skin has rough patches

_____ 8. phototherapy

H. origin and development of disease

_____ 9. seborrheic dermatitis

I. a condition caused by contact with irritants

_____ 10. xerosis

J. infection of the skin

Ⅲ. **Translate the following Chinese sentences into English.**

1. 皮肤是身体最大的器官，是一层坚固的、富有弹性的屏障，覆盖身体，保护肌肉和内部结构。

2. 诊断主要依靠典型的形态学特征、病灶的分布，以及家族和个人特异反应史。

3. 过敏性接触性皮炎是对外源性过敏原的迟发型超敏反应，而刺激物接触性皮炎是对刺激物的非特异性毒性反应。

4. 刺激物接触性皮炎在形态学上的表现与过敏性接触性皮炎类似，但通常伴有灼痛而不是瘙痒。

5. 但是，很多疾病需要全身性治疗，尤其是在病变面积较大或者局部治疗无效的情况下。

Ⅳ. **Think critically and then answer the following questions.**

1. Skin diseases usually occur in mild forms, which threaten the aesthetic look rather than the health, at least in the earlier stages. Diseases like acne and pigment disorders are treated more like a nuisance, rather than a medical condition. The cosmetic industry might make you think that a cream can best heal you and make you look beautiful. If you find a lesion on your skin, in what cases will you consult a doctor?

2. A 55-year-old man went to see the doctor, complaining of fissures and dryness of skin on the palms of his hands or the bottom of his feet. What might be the diagnosis and treatment?

Medicine in China

Appearance Anxiety

Even in the era of information overload, the Chinese have had different definitions of beauty, but the main theme revolves around two words: white and thin.

The simple and single aesthetic standard has prompted the term "appearance anxiety" to frequently top hot searches and short video platforms. A recent survey by China Youth Daily found that among females aged 18 to 35, an average of 45 minutes a day is spent looking in the mirror. For every 100 college students, 40 have undergone plastic surgery to varying degrees. Only 1 percent of the respondents said they were very satisfied with their appearance, 55 percent dissatisfied and 14 percent very dissatisfied.

The new media and the ensuing aesthetics are affecting the new generation of young people. Celebrities employ professional teams to airbrush their photos. The public has gradually become accustomed to zero-blemish skin and creamy skin so girls and women subconsciously believe that this is beautiful and it should be. They believe that the faces in the beauty cameras should be what they really look like, and they try to get closer to the illusion in real life and look at themselves with automatic filters. As a result, young women cannot bear the sight of themselves in the mirror, the real self with small acne, small freckles, and pores.

When appearance anxiety becomes severe, it may become a mental disorder or even a somatic deformity disorder. This kind of mental-psychological illness can induce depression and anxiety. In severe cases, the individual will withdraw from social interactions and may even harbor suicidal thoughts or behavior.

Exercises

Ⅰ. **Translate the underlined part into Chinese.**

Ⅱ. **Answer the following question.**

What has caused appearance anxiety among Chinese youths?

Chapter 15

Special Senses

Pre-Reading Question

What is the meaning of "see no further than one's nose"? What kind of person is one if he/she cannot see further than his/her nose?

Reading

Text A   Structure and Functions of Special Senses

The special senses include **olfaction**, taste, vision, and **audition**.

Olfaction

The **olfactory** organ is located in the mucous membrane lining the uppermost part of the roof of the nasal cavity. From the roof, the olfactory epithelium extends down both sides of the nasal cavity to cover most of the superior **concha** laterally and 1 cm of nasal septum medially. The nerve cells of the olfactory epithelium are highly sensitive to different **odors**. Olfactory neurons are continuously produced from basal cells of the olfactory epithelium and are continuously lost by the normal wear and tear process.

Olfactory neurons **project** axons to the olfactory nerve in the brain. These nerve fibers pass olfactory information to the olfactory **bulb** of the brain through **perforations** in the **cribriform** plate, which in turn projects olfactory information to the olfactory cortex and other areas. The axons from the olfactory receptors **converge** in the outer layer of the olfactory bulb within small structures called glomeruli. Mitral cells, located in the inner layer of the olfactory bulb, form synapses with the axons of the sensory neurons within glomeruli and send the information about the odor to other parts of the olfactory system (Figure 15-1).

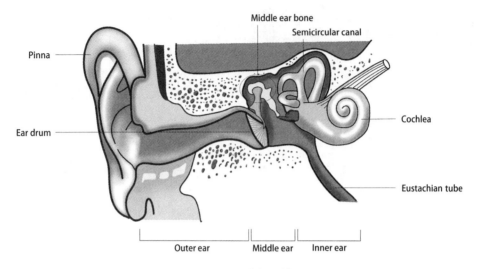

Figure 15-1   Structure of the olfactory system

Taste

The sensory organ of taste is the taste bud, which is a pale, **ovoid** structure within the **stratified** squamous epithelium. Taste buds are located on the tongue, soft palate, pharynx, larynx, epiglottis, **uvula**, and the upper one-third of the esophagus. The taste bud contains **neuroepithelial** and supporting cells. There are approximately 4 to 20 receptor cells in the center of each taste bud. The apex of each receptor cell is modified into **microvilli**, which increase the receptor surface and project into the taste pore. Receptor cells decrease in number with age.

Although man can taste a large number of substances, only four primary taste sensations are identified: sour, salty, sweet, and bitter. Most taste receptors respond to all four primary tastes but respond preferentially to only one or two.

Vision

The organ of vision is the eye; accessory structures include the eyelids, **lacrimal** glands, and the **extrinsic** eye muscles (Figure 15-2). The eye has four functional components: a protective coat, a nourishing lightproof coat, a **dioptric** system, and a **receptive** integrating layer. The protective coat is the tough, **opaque** sclera, which covers the posterior five-sixths of the eyeball; it is continuous with the **dura mater** around the **optic** nerve. The anterior one-sixth is covered by the **transparent cornea**, which belongs to the dioptric system. The nourishing coat is made up of the vascular **choroid**, which supplies nutrients to the retina and acts as a light-absorbing layer. It corresponds to the **pia-arachnoid** layer of the nervous system. Anteriorly, this coat becomes the ciliary body and iris.

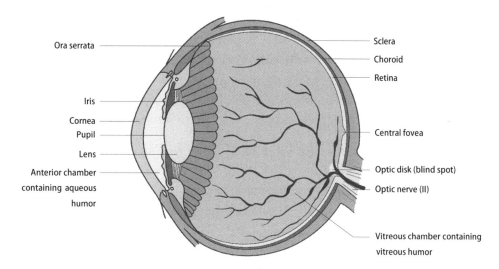

Figure 15-2   Structure of the eye

The iris ends at the pupil. The dioptric system includes the cornea, the **lens**, the **aqueous humor** within the anterior eye chamber, and the **vitreous** body. The dioptric system helps focus the image on the retina. The greatest **refraction** of incoming light takes place at the air-cornea interface.

The lens is supported by the **suspensory** ligament from the ciliary body and changes its shape to permit the change of focus. This is a function of the ciliary muscle, which is supplied by the parasympathetic nervous system.

The amount of light entering the eye is regulated by the size of the pupil. **Pupillary** size is controlled by the action of the **constrictor** and **dilator** smooth muscles of the iris. The constrictor muscle is supplied by the parasympathetic nervous system and the dilator by the sympathetic nervous system.

The receptive integrating layer is the retina. The **rods** and **cones** are the sensory retinal receptors. The rods are about 20 times as numerous as[1] the cones. The rods and cones differ in their distribution along the retina. Rods function best for peripheral vision and in dim light; cones function for central vision, in bright light, and in color **discrimination**. The outer segments of rods and cones contain the visual pigments, **rhodopsin**, and **iodopsin**, respectively.

Audition

Sound waves travel down the ear canal in the form of compression pressure waves. These pressure waves induce **deflection** of the **eardrum**, and the various structures attached to it. Part of these structures is coupled to the inner ear in a way which seems to produce an outward deflection in reaction to an inward pressure force.

The inner ear is a seashell-like **spiral** structure, in which the two chambers are separated by a thin, spiral diaphragm. Any particular acoustic signal frequency will produce a mechanical **oscillation** in the inner ear at a particular physical location. In this way, the inner ear acts as an acoustic **spectrum analyzer**, with individual **mechanoreceptors** detecting particular audio frequencies.[2] The central nervous system receives all of these signals and processes them into recognizable patterns.

The **semicircular** canals are three fluid-filled ring-like structures with hairs that are sensitive to the motion of the fluid. A **rotational acceleration** will be detected by the canals, making them useful for maintaining balance. The three canals are **oriented orthogonally** to one another, providing information about all three axes.

▶ Word Bank

olfaction /ɒl'fækʃən/ *n.* 嗅觉

olfactory /ɒl'fæktərɪ/ *a.* 嗅觉的

odor /'əʊdə/ *n.* 气味

bulb /bʌlb/ *n.* 球；球状物

cribriform /'krɪbrɪfɔːm/ *a.* 筛状的；有小孔的

ovoid /'əʊvɔɪd/ *a.* 卵形的

uvula /'juːvjʊlə/ *n.* 悬雍垂，小舌

neuroepithelial /'njʊərəʊˌepɪ'θiːlɪəl/ *a.* 神经上皮的；来自神经上皮的

microvillus /ˌmaɪkrəʊ'vɪləs/ *n.* 微绒毛（复数为 microvilli）

lacrimal /'lækrɪməl/ *a.* 泪的，泪腺的

extrinsic /eks'trɪnsɪk/ *a.* 非固有的；非本质的；外在的

dioptric /daɪ'ɒptrɪk/ *a.* 折射光学的；视力矫正用的

receptive /rɪ'septɪv/ *a.* 易接受的

dura mater /'djʊərə 'maːtə/ *n.* 硬脑膜

transparent /træns'pærənt/ *a.* 透明的；明显的

choroid /'kɔːrɔɪd/ *n.* 脉络膜

pia-arachnoid /pɪə'æræknɔɪd/ *n.* 软膜蛛网膜，柔脑脊膜

lens /lenz/ *n.* 镜片；透镜；晶体

aqueous humor /'eɪkwɪəs 'hjuːmə/ 房水，水状液

vitreous /'vɪtrɪəs/ *a.* 玻璃的；似玻璃的

suspensory /səs'pensərɪ/ *a.* 悬吊的；支持的

constrictor /kən'strɪktə/ *n.* 括约肌；压缩器

rod /rɒd/ *n.* 杆，竿

discrimination /dɪˌskrɪmɪ'neɪʃən/ *n.* 鉴赏力；辨别

iodopsin /ˌaɪə'dɒpsɪn/ *n.* 视紫蓝质，视青紫素

eardrum /'ɪədrʌm/ *n.* 耳鼓；耳膜

audition /ɔː'dɪʃən/ *n.* 听；听力

concha /'kɒŋkə/ *n.* 鼻甲

project /prə'dʒekt/ *v.* 投射；突出

perforation /ˌpɜːfə'reɪʃən/ *n.* 孔

converge /kən'vɜːdʒ/ *v.* 聚合，集中

stratify /'strætɪfaɪ/ *v.* 分层，成层

opaque /əʊ'peɪk/ *a.* 不透明的

optic /'ɒptɪk/ *a.* 视觉的；光学的

cornea /'kɔːnɪə/ *n.* 角膜

refraction /rɪ'frækʃən/ *n.* 折光，折射

pupillary /'pʊpɪlərɪ/ *a.* 瞳孔的

dilator /daɪ'leɪtə/ *n.* 扩张肌；扩张器

cone /kəʊn/ *n.* 圆锥体；锥形物；球果

rhodopsin /rəʊ'dɒpsɪn/ *n.* 视紫质，视网膜紫质

deflection /dɪ'flekʃən/ *n.* 歪斜；偏向；偏转角

spiral /'spaɪrəl/ *a.* 螺旋的；螺旋状的

oscillation /ˌɒsɪ'leɪʃən/ *n.* 振动；振幅

analyzer /'ænəˌlaɪzə/ *n.* 分析仪；分析者

mechanoreceptor /ˌmekəˌnəʊrɪ'septə/ *n.* 机械性刺激感受器；机械敏感性受体

semicircular /ˌsemɪ'sɜːkjʊlə/ *a.* 半圆的

acceleration /əkˌselə'reɪʃən/ *n.* 加速

orthogonally /ɔː'θɒɡənlɪ/ *ad.* 直角地，直交地，正交地

spectrum /'spektrəm/ *n.* 幅度；范围；光谱；频谱

rotational /rəʊ'teɪʃənəl/ *a.* 回转的；轮流的

orient /'ɔːrɪənt/ *v.* 确定方向；适应

▶ Notes

1. times as many/numerous as 是固定搭配，意为是……的……倍。如：If the global climate becomes 2 degrees warmer, there will be about 10 times as many extreme storm surges.（如果全球气候变暖 2℃，极端风暴潮的数量将为 10 倍。）

2. 该句中含有 with 引导的独立主格结构，在句中作伴随状语。在此独立主格中，individual mechanoreceptors 是现在分词 detecting 的逻辑主语。

Exercises

Ⅰ. **Choose the best answer to each of the following questions.**

1. Where is the olfactory organ located?
   A. In the mucous membrane.　　　　　B. In the superior concha.
   C. In the nasal cavity.　　　　　　　D. In the nasal septum.

2. Why do the elderly tend to be insensitive to odors?
   A. Because their olfactory nerves are insensitive to different odors.
   B. Because their olfactory neurons are continuously lost due to normal wear.
   C. Because their olfactory neurons become weak as they age.
   D. Because their olfactory neurons are affected by tears.

3. Which of the following statements describes the sensory organ correctly?
   A. Taste bud is the major sensory organ of taste.
   B. The tongue is the major sensory organ of taste.
   C. The sensory organ of taste is located on the tongue.
   D. The function of the sensory organ of taste will not decline with age.

4. Which of the following is NOT true about taste?
   A. One can taste many substances.
   B. One can identify four main tastes.
   C. Taste sensations differ from person to person.
   D. Most taste receptors respond to the four main tastes equally.

5. What is the function of the protective coat of the eye?
    A. Protecting the tough opaque sclera.
    B. Providing nutrients for the eyeball.
    C. Protecting the inner structure of the eye.
    D. Protecting the eyeball.

6. Which of the following serves as the nourishing coat of the eye?
    A. The sclera.   B. The iris.
    C. The cornea.   D. The retina.

7. What role does the nervous system play in vision?
    A. The parasympathetic nervous system controls the ciliary muscle.
    B. The parasympathetic nervous system enlarges the size of the pupil.
    C. The sympathetic nervous system reduces the size of the pupil.
    D. The sympathetic nervous system helps focus the image on the retina.

8. Which of the following statement correctly describes the rods and cones in the retina?
    A. They receive and integrate lights.
    B. They are evenly distributed.
    C. They function best on sunny days.
    D. They function best on gloomy days.

9. What is the function of the inner ear?
    A. Inducing deflection of the eardrum.
    B. Producing mechanical oscillation.
    C. Analyzing acoustic spectrum.
    D. Processing sound signals.

10. Which of the following statements describes the function of semicircular canals?
    A. They are the canals through which sound waves travel.
    B. They can detect the motion of the fluid.
    C. They help to maintain balance.
    D. They support the inner ear.

Ⅱ. **Group the following organs into the major categories they belong to.**

epiglottis, esophagus, glomeruli, larynx, mitral cells, olfactory bulb, olfactory epithelium, pharynx, soft palate, superior concha, uvula

The olfaction system: _____

_____

The taste system: _____

_____

III . Fill in each blank in the following paragraph with a word in the box. Change the form of words if necessary.

absence	presence	loud	deafness	impairment
increase	insensitivity	complete	voice	production
sensitivity	severity	decrease	disease	whole

Hearing loss is a partial or total inability to hear. Hearing loss exists when there is diminished 1_____ to the sounds normally heard. The term hearing 2_____ is usually reserved for people who have relative 3_____ to sound in the speech frequencies. The 4_____ of hearing loss is categorized according to the 5_____ in volume above the usual level before the listener can detect it. 6_____ is defined as a degree of impairment such that a person is unable to understand speech even in the 7_____ of an amplifier (扩音器). In profound deafness, even the 8_____ sounds produced by an amplifier may not be detected. In 9_____ deafness, no sounds at all, regardless of amplification or method of 10_____ , are heard.

IV. Translate the following English sentences into Chinese.

1. Olfactory neurons are continuously produced from basal cells of the olfactory epithelium and are continuously lost by the normal wear and tear process.

2. These nerve fibers pass olfactory information to the olfactory bulb of the brain through perforations in the cribriform plate, which in turn projects olfactory information to the olfactory cortex and other areas.

3. The lens is supported by the suspensory ligament from the ciliary body and changes its shape to permit the change of focus.

4. Part of these structures is coupled to the inner ear in a way which seems to produce an outward deflection in reaction to an inward pressure force.

5. A rotational acceleration will be detected by the canals, making them useful for maintaining balance.

Ⅳ. **Write a 100-word summary of the four functional components of the eye and their functions.**

Reading

Text B   Diseases of Special Senses and Their Treatment

Cataract

Cataract is the leading cause of blindness and visual loss in the world. The great majority of cases represent normal aging changes in which progressive yellowing of the lens nucleus and **hydration** of the lens cortex are seen. **Prolonged** exposure to ultraviolet radiation has been shown to be the major cause. Surgical **extraction** is required to improve vision; however, there is no known medical treatment.

Nearly all patients older than 50 demonstrate some degree of degenerative lens changes. Visual disability depends on the extent of **lenticular** changes as well as on the visual demands of the patient. Very rarely is cataract extraction medically indicated. Mature, swollen cataracts may induce **glaucoma** by narrowing the anterior chamber angle. **Hypermature**, **liquefied** cataracts may leak lens protein and thereby cause **uveitis**. In the majority of cases, however, elective cataract extraction serves to restore lost vision. There is no urgency in most cases, and patients who are told they must have cataract surgery in the absence of[1] disabling visual complaints should **beware**.

Congenital cataracts may be associated with metabolic disease, result from **intrauterine** TORCH[2] infections, or be **familial**. Traumatic cataracts result from hydration after **penetrating** injury to the lens. Some cataracts may be characteristic in color or location, such as the sunflower cataract of Wilson's disease[3] or the posterior **subcapsular** cataract often resulting from systemic corticosteroid use.

Cataract extraction with **intraocular** lens implantation has become a very successful procedure in the developed world. Potential complications include **cystoid macular** edema, **astigmatism**, **retinal detachment**, and **endophthalmitis**. Current methods of surgery include small, **self-sealing incisions** performed under local or topical anesthesia. Prognosis for visual recovery is excellent.

Disorders of Smell and Taste

The senses of taste and smell are very closely related. Some people who go to the doctor because they think they have lost their sense of taste are surprised to learn that they have a smell disorder instead.

The most common taste disorder is **phantom** taste perception; that is, a **lingering**, often unpleasant taste even though you have nothing in your mouth. We also can experience a reduced ability to taste sweet, sour, bitter, salty, or **umami**, a condition called **hypogeusia**. Some people cannot detect any taste, which is called **ageusia**. True taste loss, however, is rare. Most often, people are experiencing a loss of smell instead of a loss of taste.

In other disorders of the chemical senses, an odor, a taste, or a flavor may be distorted. **Dysgeusia** is a condition in which a **foul**, salty, **rancid**, or **metallic** taste sensation will persist in the mouth. Dysgeusia is sometimes accompanied by burning mouth syndrome, a condition in which a person experiences a painful burning sensation in the mouth. Although it can affect anyone, burning mouth syndrome is most common in middle-aged and older women.

Loss of taste and smell can create serious health issues. Disorders of taste interfere with digestion because taste stimulation alters salivary and pancreatic flow, gastric contractions, and intestinal **motility**. Smell also contributes to the **ingestion** of food because much of what is tasted derives from olfactory stimulation during ingestion and chewing. An inability to detect **noxious** tastes and odors can result in food or gas poisoning, particularly in elderly people. In extreme cases, **chemosensory** disorders can lead to overwhelming stress, **anorexia**, and depression.

The most frequently encountered causes of loss of smell are local obstructive disease, viral infections, head injuries, and normal aging. Patients can lose their sense of smell not only from chronic allergies and sinusitis but also from the nasal **sprays** and **drops** that they use to treat these conditions. The most common causes of loss of the sense of taste are viral infections and drug ingestion, particularly **antirheumatic** and **antiproliferative** drugs. Disturbances of smell and taste in **malnourished** patients may be due to specific deficiencies in vitamins and minerals, such as zinc. Viral illnesses such as influenza and viral hepatitis produce disorders in both taste and smell. **Multifocal** neurologic disorders such as multiple sclerosis can affect the central olfactory and **gustatory** pathways at multiple levels; as a result, abnormalities of taste and smell are common in such patients.

Treatment of olfactory **dysfunction** is aimed at opening the air passageways while preserving the olfactory epithelium. **Intranasal** steroids, antibiotics, and allergic therapies are useful in selected cases.

Hearing Loss

Hearing loss, or deafness, can be present at birth (congenital), or become evident later in life (acquired). The distinction between acquired and congenital deafness specifies only the time when the deafness appears. It does not specify whether the cause of the deafness is genetic (inherited).

Acquired deafness may or may not be genetic. For example, it may be a manifestation of a delayed-onset form of genetic deafness. Alternatively, acquired deafness may result from damage to the ear due to noise or from other conditions.

Similarly, congenital deafness may or may not be genetic. For example, it may be associated with a white **forelock**, and be caused by a genetic disease called **Waardenburg syndrome**[4]. In fact, more than half of congenital hearing loss is inherited. Alternatively, congenital deafness may be due to a condition or infection to which the mother was exposed during pregnancy, such as the **rubella** virus.

Symptoms of hearing loss include mild loss of high-frequency hearing, hearing loss associated with ringing or noises (**tinnitus**), and complete deafness. Symptoms may develop gradually over time with many causes of hearing loss.

People who are experiencing hearing loss may refrain from[5] taking part in conversations, may turn the volume up high on the radio or TV, and may frequently ask others to repeat what they have said.

The treatment of hearing loss depends on its cause. For example, ear wax can be removed; ear infections can be treated with medications; diseases that cause inflammation of the ear can be treated with medication; medications that are toxic to the ear can be avoided; and occasionally surgical procedures are necessary.

▶ Word Bank

cataract /'kætərækt/ *n.* 白内障

prolonged /prə'lɒŋd/ *a.* 持续很久的

lenticular /len'tɪkjʊlə/ *a.* 透镜状的；两面凸的；晶状体的

glaucoma /glɔː'kəʊmə/ *n.* 青光眼

liquefy /'lɪkwɪfaɪ/ *v.* 液化

beware /bɪ'weə/ *v.* 小心，谨防

familial /fə'mɪliəl/ *a.* 家庭的；家族遗传的

subcapsular /sʌb'kæpsjʊlə/ *a.* 囊下的

cystoid /'sɪstɔɪd/ *a.* 囊样的；似膀胱的

astigmatism /ə'stɪɡmə͵tɪzəm/ *n.* 散光

detachment /dɪ'tætʃmənt/ *n.* 脱离

self-sealing /'self'siːlɪŋ/ *a.* 自动封口的，自动密封的

phantom /'fæntəm/ *a.* 错觉的；幻影的；幽灵的

umami /uː'mɑːmɪ/ *n.* 鲜味

hydration /haɪ'dreɪʃən/ *n.* 水合作用

extraction /ɪk'strækʃən/ *n.* 抽出；拔出；抽出物

hypermature /͵haɪpəmə'tjʊə/ *a.* 过成熟的

uveitis /͵juːvɪ'aɪtɪs/ *n.* 眼色素层炎，葡萄膜炎

intrauterine /͵ɪntrə'juːtərɪn/ *a.* 子宫内的

penetrate /'penɪtreɪt/ *v.* 穿透

intraocular /͵ɪntrə'ɒkjʊlə/ *a.* 眼内的

macular /'mækjʊlə/ *a.* 有斑点的；有污点的

retinal /'retɪnəl/ *a.* 视网膜的

endophthalmitis /͵endəfθəl'maɪtɪs/ *n.* 眼内炎

incision /ɪn'sɪʒən/ *n.* 切口；切割

linger /'lɪŋɡə/ *v.* 拖延；逗留

hypogeusia /͵haɪpə'dʒuːʒə/ *n.* 味觉减退，味觉迟钝

ageusia /eɪˈgjuːzɪə/ *n.* 味觉丧失

dysgeusia /dɪsˈdʒuːzɪə/ *n.* 味觉倒错，味觉障碍

foul /faʊl/ *a.* 恶臭的，污秽的

rancid /ˈrænsɪd/ *a.* 有腐臭油脂味的，令人作呕的

metallic /mɪˈtælɪk/ *a.* 金属的

motility /məʊˈtɪlɪtɪ/ *n.* 运动性；自动力

noxious /ˈnɒkʃəs/ *a.* 有害的，有毒的

chemosensory /ˌkeməʊˈsensərɪ/ *a.* 化学感应的

anorexia /ˌænəˈreksɪə/ *n.* 厌食症

spray /spreɪ/ *n.* 喷雾；喷雾器

drop /drɒp/ *n.* 滴；微量；滴状物

antirheumatic /ˌæntɪruːˈmætɪk/ *n.* 抗风湿药

antiproliferative /ˌæntiprəˈlɪfərətɪv/ *a.* 抗增殖的

malnourish /mælˈnʌrɪʃ/ *v.* 营养不良

multifocal /ˌmʌltɪˈfəʊkəl/ *a.* 多病灶的

gustatory /ˈgʌstəˌtərɪ/ *a.* 味觉的

dysfunction /dɪsˈfʌŋkʃən/ *n.* 功能不良，机能障碍

intranasal /ˌɪntrəˈneɪzəl/ *a.* 鼻内的

forelock /ˈfɔːlɒk/ *n.* 额发，额毛

Waardenburg syndrome /ˈwɔː dənbəg ˈsɪndrəʊm/ 瓦登伯格氏症候群

rubella /ruːˈbelə/ *n.* 风疹

tinnitus /tɪˈnaɪtɪs/ *n.* 耳鸣

▶ Notes

1.　该句中 in the absence of 意思为缺乏，不存在。现在分词 disabling 作定语，意思为使失去能力的，致残的。

2.　TORCH 指一组病原体：T 指 toxoplasma（弓形体），O 指 others（其他），比如乙型肝炎病毒、HIV 病毒、梅毒螺旋体等，R 指 rubella virus（风疹病毒），C 指 cytomegalovirus（巨细胞病毒），H 指 herpes virus（疱疹病毒）。TORCH 系列中的几种微生物都可通过胎盘影响胎儿早期的正常发育，并引起多种先天性疾病，因此检测 TORCH 病毒感染常作为妇女怀孕期生殖道感染的常规检查项目。

3.　sunflower cataract 指向日葵状白内障。Wilson's disease 译为威尔森病，是一种先天性代谢疾病，特点是无法将体内的铜质正常代谢，造成过多铜离子在肝脏及脑部等器官堆积沉淀，从而造成多种病变。

4.　Waardenburg syndrome 瓦登伯革氏症候群，是神经色素细胞移行异常所导致的疾病，又称"蓝眼珠宝宝"。该病患者除了眼珠因色素较少呈天蓝色外，在额头常有一小撮白发。

5.　refrain from 为固定搭配，意为克制，避免。如：We refrained from talking until we knew that it was safe.（我们缄默不语，直到确定安全了才开始说话。）。

Exercises

Ⅰ. **For each of the following statements, write "T" if the statement is true and "F" if the statement is false in the blank.**

_____ 1.　Cataracts can be treated both medically and surgically.

_____ 2. Degenerative changes of the lens occur in most people above 50 years with cataracts.

_____ 3. Most patients with cataracts should receive cataract extraction once the cataract is diagnosed.

_____ 4. Some people may actually suffer loss of smell when they cannot taste any flavor.

_____ 5. Burning mouth syndrome is sometimes accompanied by taste distortion.

_____ 6. Loss of taste can definitely lead to anorexia, particularly in elderly people.

_____ 7. Deficiency of zinc may lead to disorders of smell and taste.

_____ 8. Acquired deafness is not inherited.

_____ 9. Congenital deafness may also be caused by the mother's infection during pregnancy.

_____ 10. Patients suffering from hearing loss may not be as sociable as people with normal hearing.

Ⅱ. **Match each term in Column A with its correct description in Column B. Write the corresponding letter in the blank.**

Column A	Column B
_____ 1. ageusia	A. a disease involving the opacification（浑浊化）of the natural lens of the eye
_____ 2. cataract	B. a disease that damages the optic nerve and impairs vision
_____ 3. dysgeusia	C. within the eyeball
_____ 4. deafness	D. a condition in which patients have reduced ability to taste tastes
_____ 5. genetic deafness	E. a condition in which the patient cannot detect any taste
_____ 6. glaucoma	F. a condition with strange taste sensation persisting in the mouth
_____ 7. hypogeusia	G. complete or partial loss of the ability to hear

_____ 8. tinnitus   H. a type of hearing loss associated with ringing or noises

_____ 9. intraocular   I. a soft yellow wax secreted by glands in the ear canal

_____ 10. ear wax   J. inherited deafness caused by genetic changes

Ⅲ. **Translate the following Chinese sentences into English.**

1. 大多数白内障都是由于年龄增长引起晶状体核发生进行性变黄以及晶状体皮质水合。

2. 先天性白内障可能与代谢疾病有关，也可能由子宫内的 TORCH 感染引起或是由家族遗传的。

3. 嗅觉也影响食物的摄入，因为人们品尝到的味道源于摄入和咀嚼食物时的嗅觉刺激。

4. 先天性听力丧失和后天性听力丧失的区别仅在于其发病时间不同。

5. 遭受听力丧失的人可能会避免与人交谈，或将收音机或电视机的音量调高，或不断让别人重复说过的话。

Ⅳ. **Think critically and then answer the following questions.**

1. Is loss of taste and smell normal with aging, or could loss of taste and smell have other causes? If one suffers from such a condition, what advice will you give him or her?

2. Does listening to music at low volume levels, but for 5–6 hours or more every day, make tinnitus worse? Is it better to listen via speakers or headphones?

Medicine in China

Auricular Healthcare in TCM

Traditional Chinese Medicine (TCM) is a great treasure, in which traditional auricular massage for health-keeping is an important component and a precious heritage. Traditional auricular massage for health-keeping, as an essential part of traditional "ear therapy", has been not only historically long-standing and well established but also greatly beneficial for the public to build body and prolong lives.

The origin and testimony of the enduring scientific property and rationality of auricular healthcare massage can be verified in Chinese medical classics of all historical times. For instance, *The Moxibustion Classic of Eleven Meridians of Yin-yang (Yinyang Shiyimai Jiujing)*, one of the earliest medical works that existed in China, was unearthed from No. 3 Mawangdui Tomb of Han Dynasty in 1973 in Changsha, Hunan province. It was recorded in this book "an 'ear meridian' originates from the back of hands and ascends up to the inside of the ear".

In later generations, auricular healthcare massage was increasingly adored and popularized by TCM physicians with the purpose of strengthening body building, preventing and curing diseases, and furthermore prolonging lives. Besides, in the practice of cultivation and healthcare, they also summed up some proverbs of auricular healthcare such as "ears should be pressed often" and "ears should be frequently flicked". In addition, Taoism that advocated health cultivation also paid much attention to auricular healthcare and massage. TCM classics and Taoism have recorded a lot of traditional auricular healthcare methods which were created, practiced and inherited based on the plain understanding of close relations between the auricle and human body, and viscera.

Exercises

Ⅰ. **Translate the underlined part into Chinese.**

Ⅱ. **Answer the following question.**

What is the wisdom embodied in TCM's auricular healthcare?